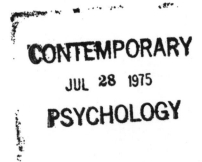

CONTEMPORARY

PSYCHOLOGY

JON ALAN KANGAS, Ph.D., is a clinical psychologist and Director of the Testing and Counseling Center at the University of Santa Clara. Graduating Summa Cum Laude from Fresno State College, he went on to obtain his masters and doctoral degrees from Washington State University. A humanist at heart, his current interest is in psychosynthesis, integrating transactional, analytic, gestalt, and bioenergetic approaches to growth.

GEORGE FREEMAN SOLOMON, M.D., is Clinical Professor of Psychiatry at UCLA, Director of Medical Education of the Fresno County Department of Health, and Chief of Psychiatry at Valley Medical Center of Fresno. He is the author of fifty articles and has recently developed a unique model treatment unit for criminal offenders through his work in the psychodynamics of violence and antisocial behavior.

# Jon Alan Kangas
# George Freeman Solomon

# THE PSYCHOLOGY
# OF
# STRENGTH

A SPECTRUM BOOK

PRENTICE-HALL, INC., Englewood Cliffs, New Jersey

*Library of Congress Cataloging in Publication Data*

KANGAS, JON ALAN.
  The psychology of strength.

  (A Spectrum Book)
  Bibliography: p.
  1. Emotional maturity.  2. Mental hygiene.
I. Solomon, George F., joint author.  II. Title.
[DNLM:  1. Emotions.  2. Mental health.  WM75 K16p]
BF710.K36        155.2'5        75-2212
ISBN 0-13-736637-X
ISBN 0-13-736629-9 pbk.

BF710
K36

10 9 8 7 6 5 4 3 2 1

PRENTICE-HALL INTERNATIONAL, INC. *(London)*
PRENTICE-HALL OF AUSTRALIA PTY. LTD. *(Sydney)*
PRENTICE-HALL OF CANADA LTD. *(Toronto)*
PRENTICE-HALL OF INDIA PRIVATE LIMITED *(New Delhi)*
PRENTICE-HALL OF JAPAN, INC. *(Tokyo)*
PRENTICE-HALL OF SOUTHEAST ASIA (PTE.) LTD. *(Singapore)*

*To our mentors in humanistic psychology and in psychoanalysis, deceased and living: Abraham Maslow and Sigmund Freud; Alan Button and Joseph C. Solomon.*

# CONTENTS

# PREFACE

This book is the outgrowth of a short article of the same title abstracted and reported in a number of newspapers and magazines, including *America*, the Jesuit magazine. Our co-author in the original manuscript was K. Michael Schmidt, Ph.D., former director of the Counseling and Testing Center, University of Santa Clara, for whose support and suggestions we are indebted. We were encouraged by a number of readers to expand the original brief paper, characterizing the strong person and outlining his problems, into a broader discussion of the nature, achievement, and consequences of psychological strength.

This book represents the collaboration of a humanistically oriented psychologist and a psychoanalytically and biologically oriented psychiatrist. We have attempted to be understandable to a broad range of readers, since we feel everyone has the capacity for growth and enhanced strength. This book makes no pretense of being a scholarly or scientific treatise, which both authors are accustomed to preparing in other contexts, but rather is very much a personal expression. Also, even though we have found our own conceptions of psychological strength to be generally helpful, we in no way assume their universality. Because of the limitations in our own knowledge and perspective, we have sought the valuable collaboration of others.

Brian Thorvaldson, a perceptive young student of psychology at the University of Hawaii, has provided us with general criticisms, useful interpretations of strength, and especially with speculations about future potentialities for human development. Patricia Howe is a partner of L. F. Rothschild and Co. and a member of the New York Stock Exchange. Her achievements in competitive business, combined with a firm sense of feminine identity, put her in a unique position to comment on the difficult and fluid subject of strength and femininity. Diana Bunce, lovely wife of an ex-football star, now medical student, has had the frequent experience of being reacted to for her striking appearance and the glamorous status of her husband, and is keenly aware of the issues facing the intelligent, attractive, feminine young woman. In this regard, as well as many others, we must also cite the advice and support of our wives, Anne and Gabriella. The ego psychological concepts of Joseph C. Solomon, M.D., father of the second author, recur throughout the book. Ruth Freeman Solomon, mother of George F. Solomon and author of several successful novels, gave valuable editorial advice. Muriel Jeffrey and Elizabeth Yegan provided valuable technical assistance. We are particularly grateful for the skilled editorial assistance of our publisher.

A nagging semantic problem troubled us throughout the writing. There is no English pronoun to express "he or she." We were tempted to neologize with "hs" but generally settled for the unsatisfactory convention of utilizing "he" or "his" to refer to attributes applicable to either sex. We do not intend this to be a book about the strong man but rather about the strong person. We specifically differentiate in the few instances when masculinity or femininity *per se* is discussed. We cannot deny, however, that as men, even with the aid of our female collaborators, we cannot completely escape from our own inevitable male bias any more than we can totally avoid our cultural ones. We try to speak directly and personally to the reader and thus do not worry about the grammar of the "impersonal you" that our eighth grade teachers bade us avoid. (After all, the strong person is unlikely to be overly bound by convention!)

Clinical illustrations are highly disguised to protect individuals except ourselves.

# INTRODUCTION

Man is limited by the conceptions or the "cosmology" defining himself, his potentialities, and his personal world, as provided by his culture or chosen by himself from the range of which he is aware. Limiting self-conceptions retard growth. The attractive woman who perceives herself as ugly because she had been an awkward, overweight child tends to behave as though she were unattractive or needs continually to reassure herself about her attractiveness. The man of deep resources who sees himself as relatively incompetent does not undertake something of which he is capable. On the other hand, grandiose conceptions of one's strength and potentiality can lead a man to lose sight of his personal reality and to overwhelm his resources. However, the "great man"—or woman—is generally the one who has turned seemingly grandiose fantasies into reality. The pursuit of illusionary images of strength may occupy a person for a lifetime. When fantasied goals are substituted for genuine fulfillment or are attempts to compensate for basic unmet needs and feelings of inadequacy, unworthiness, or emptiness, they often fail to satisfy or unify. The fame, wealth, glamor, and adulation of the movie or pop star do not always prevent despair, addiction, or suicide.

As each man attempts to align himself more harmoniously with his personal cosmos, as he tries to find a more peaceful life within, as he tries to reduce the dissonance he feels in relationship to others, as he seeks to lessen the need to contend with himself, others, and the world, he finds himself, for better or worse, a conceptual animal. His conceptions can either lead or mislead him in his attempts to live a more peaceful and fulfilling existence. Conceptualizations of strength, goals, and values are ultimately only guides to enriched experience. As concepts and abstractions, they are not experience itself. As guides, they are in themselves not true or false, they are only useful to a greater or lesser degree. Persons starting from different levels of experience and understanding may need different guides to lead the way. The finest desert guide may not be of much use on the mountain. A man who is hungry may need to learn how to work and acquire food. A man secure in his basic needs may need to meditate and search within for greater peace. A particular conception of strength may lead one person forward, frustrate and confuse another, and even cause a third to regress.

Our attempt in the next several chapters is to provide another guide, another way of conceptualizing strength, that we hope will aid the reader in experiencing greater levels of personal integration and personal harmony by altering his path slightly, by changing his perceptions in a way that will enhance the reader's ability to tap his own personal reservoirs of strength. Our conceptions of strength will undoubtedly be overwhelming for some and will be inadequate for others. Our hope is that they may provide a step forward for many.

Thus, ours is a book about emotional health. There is a vast literature concerned with psychopathology, little about psychic well-being. We conceive psychological disturbances to be a result of relative failure in psychological development and of efforts to repair or secondarily to master those failures. In order to move toward greater health, one must be able to conceive of a direction of growth as a prerequisite to its accomplishment. Culturally, our own growth has been limited by traditional and conventional views of the nature of psychological strength and by stereotyped models or ego ideals. There has been a dearth of new models of strength appropriate to our complex, changing, and heterogeneous contemporary society. Our book is an attempt to fill this void by providing a workable framework by which to approach fulfillment of human potential in our culture.

Most dynamic psychologies, including those of Freud, Sullivan, Erikson, Piaget, and Maslow, have a developmental frame of reference. Our book emerges from this tradition and draws primarily from a humanistic perspective, though it also encompasses psychoanalytic and ego psychology. Growth and maturation entail biological, social, and intrapsychic processes. For Freud, mature man was a "genital character," whose adult heterosexual orientation incorporated and subordinated pregenital components. Erikson places mutuality at the developmental summit. Joseph Solomon sees each age of man as presenting developmental tasks to be mastered with specific personality traits arising from successful mastery or from secondary reparative attempts at integration, winding up with serenity as a trait characteristic of successful old age. Maslow sees self-actualization as a process attained through successful prior meeting of lower order needs.

We, too, feel that the organism has an intrinsic tendency toward health and healing, psychological as well as physical, and toward reaching higher levels of integration. The elimination of extrinsic or intrinsic blocks to growth permits movement toward fulfillment and actualization. Man cannot grow if coerced by an oppressive society; if basic needs, emotional or economic, remain unmet; if oppressed and imprisoned by internalized conflicts or commands from his own past; or if ignorant of what constitutes health and human potential. This book attempts to define specific aspects of psychological health, strength, and potentiality in an effort to overcome the ignorance that can block development. Political and economic action and psychotherapeutic intervention are necessary to overcome the other obstacles to development.

We hope to help the reader in his or her quest for greater strength and for further growth. We also hope to help strong persons deal with problems unique to strength. The reader will be disappointed, however, if he or she expects to find out what the strong person *is,* for there are multiple paths to greater strength and a host of ways in which psychological strength is expressed.

There is no such being as *the* strong person. Strength is better described in terms of process than as a state. There are a variety of ways in which psychological strength is expressed. One is strong at a given time, in relation to a specific situation or to a particular person. Overall psychological strength is expressed in three fundamental areas: one's relationship to oneself and one's inner world; one's relationship to others and capacity for intimacy; and one's ability to handle stress and challenges in the real world. Strength, thus, has aspects of inner, interpersonal, and outer mastery.

Strength is exhibited in the act of a person's choosing: to be or to do that which is best for himself and others in a given situation; that which results in the greater inner personal harmony; that which aligns him and others most successfully with each other; that which results in lessened dissonance with the world. We feel that an essence of strength is the ability to choose, implying the possibility of free will. Even the words we use to describe this process are in their very nature static and analytical and, as such, cannot do justice to all the variables involved in the act of choice. Yet, just as maps are not the terrain, they can still be helpful.

What man's full and ultimate potential may be is beyond our personal experience, although we attempt to capture glimpses of it. Some say that man's potential has already been demonstrated and made known in the person of Jesus Christ, or Mohammed, Buddha, or others. Indeed, examples set by prophets, saints, and lesser but still powerful men *do* indicate the potentials within man for developing his strength. If such men have reached the top of a ladder leading to "harmony with the universe," "oneness with God," "the fulfillment of human potential," or all of the preceding, then our conceptions may be designed to help persons climb to some intermediate rung.

# PART ONE:

## Notions of Strength

# 1

# PSEUDO-STRENGTH

The strong person. Visions of Prince Valiant, Alexander the Great, Spartacus, early Christians facing lions, Socrates in his Academy, Nathan Hale, Albert Schweitzer, John Glenn, Evel Knievel all flash to mind, coloring our personal images of strength. Varying from one time to another, one land to the next, cultural ego-ideals typically epitomize important aspects of strength. When accepted as portraying all that is strength, these notions limit and restrict our vision and in turn our potential for strength. They become static, inviting images of strength, like Sirens to Homer, enticing but deadly.

Because your self-esteem, for example, is likely to be inversely proportional to the difference between your actual self-concept and your ideal self-concept (ego-ideal), it is understandable how an ego-ideal that is limiting, unrealistically lofty, or distorted can have direct consequences on your mental health. So, even though we cannot explore all the major historical and contemporary cross-cultural images of strength (typically the strong *man*), we do want to provide a sampling of some of the more prevalent idealized notions of strength.

Our own conception of psychological strength encompasses mastery of inner, interpersonal, and outer dimensions. Most limiting notions of strength tend to be extreme examples of one or another of these aspects of strength at the expense of one or both of the other dimensions. So great may a person's strength be in one area that the severe limitations in the others may not be readily apparent. Such a pseudo-strong person, epitomizing one aspect of strength, may easily be idealized as *the* model of strength. But in modeling oneself after such a person, one tends to inherit the same unseen limitations as the idol.

The strong person, or more accurately and in keeping with the basic stance of this book, the person who consistently behaves in strong ways, cannot always be discerned solely by his actions. Similar behaviors, even socially desirable ones, may have different inner meanings. For example, generosity, a "good" trait, can emerge as an expression of inner bountifulness stemming from having oneself been a recipient of generosity and kindness or, on the other hand, can arise in the service of defenses: to deny one's acquisitive wishes, to foster identification with the recipient in the face of an actual wish to receive rather than to give, to meet power needs by enabling one to become head of a charitable organization or to acquire praise or prestige. The behavior itself does not necessarily convey its motivations or its roots. It is thus a tricky business to quickly assess the strength of another. It is also for this very reason that many of us, judging the strength of others by their actions, may emulate those who appear to be strong, but who in fact may fall in the ranks of the apparently or pseudo-strong.

### Strength as Mastery

Primary mastery refers to the successful accomplishment of a developmental task or the meeting of an environmental challenge leading to resolution, growth, and absence of residual conflict. Defenses or secondary masteries (secondary integrations) are attempts at repair or healing of conflicts not initially overcome and, as such, bear the scars of the original wounds. Scar tissue is rarely as strong or resilient as the original healthy tissue, though it does serve an important purpose and may allow apparently normal function under most circumstances. To give another physiological analogy, we might cite the compensation of the heart in the face of a cardiovascular defect. The heart muscle has a capacity to enlarge (hypertrophy) and thus pump more strongly when there is a leaky valve or high blood pressure. Up to a point, this hypertrophy can maintain the circulation under normal circumstances. The individual appears to be functioning quite adequately and may be unaware of any deficiency. He has limited reserves, however, in the face of special demands, high levels of effort or stress, under which circumstances cardiac decompensation or heart failure can set in. Likewise, the individual possessing many traits and adaptations based on defensive operations, which ward off anxieties and fears from the past or help adapt to a world misperceived through distortions based on idiosyncratic earlier experience, has lessened psychological reserve. Though such an individual may be compensated in the sense that there is no manifest anxiety, depression, or alienation under most circumstances, psychopathological states in terms of uncomfortable, inappropriate feelings and/or neurotic symptoms may readily ensue in situations of high demand or stress. Indeed, psychological strength, closely related to the concept of "ego strength" in the psychoanalytic frame of reference, can be thought of as the sum of one's primary masteries minus the sum of one's secondary masteries, or, more simply, as the sum of one's victories minus the sum of one's defeats. Obviously, in these terms, a person is relatively weak if there are either too few victories or too many defeats. Both the person who has been overwhelmed by harsh circumstances beyond his capacity to cope or the one who has been overprotected and sheltered from the vicissitudes of life are likely to be weak or to have characteristics of what we term pseudo-strength rather than of genuine strength.

With these comments in mind let us proceed to identify some of these historical and contemporary models and notions of strength that are inviting but narrow and tend to block development, keeping in mind that without a balance and integration of inner mastery, interpersonal competence, and outer mastery, full psychological strength is not achieved.

## OUTER MASTERY

### *Physical Strength and Power*

Obviously, sheer physical prowess is the most primitive form of personal strength. The dominant male in a primate troop is generally the largest and strongest, although often also the most wily. The caricature of the caveman dragging off his "bride" by the hair comes to mind. With the advent of tools and increasing social complexity, intelligence and leadership skills became more important than brute strength. Derivatives of the archetypal prowess model persist in the glorification of power and the powerful. Individually, the power-seeking or grandiose person has often been the victim of profound feelings of childhood helplessness and unimportance. Culturally, deification of power may be seen as a defense against man's basic vulnerability and frailty. As Erich Fromm has pointed out, weaker individuals will often abrogate their own freedom for the false security of protection by a powerful leader. Such protection may at one time have had a more realistic basis, as, for example, the vassal under the shelter of the lord and his castle. Trappings of power serve to induce awe of the leader. The planes, helicopters, fancy-dress guards, and country estates of presidents seem to function as did the gilded carriages, household cavalry, and castles of kings. The social bonds based upon power are intrinsically more fragile than those based upon affection and mutual regard. The soldier loyal to his comrades and lieutenant fights harder than the one coerced, who may turn against the leader (as in the "fragging" by unmotivated, resentful soldiers in Vietnam).

### Heroics versus Heroism

While the power-seeking and the manipulative attempt to change the behavior of others in order to be in control, some seek to prove strength by continual demonstrations of prowess or bravery. While outwardly reflecting strength, heroics, unlike heroism, do not reflect inner strength, but rather are a way to compensate for basic feelings of vulnerability or fearfulness. Those asked to name strong persons often point to heroes, men or women of valor and courage—for example, the war hero who threw a live grenade from the bunker, the cop who crawled out on a ledge to bring in the suicidal woman, the housewife who rushed into a burning building to rescue children. Which of these acts is a symbol of inner strength and which reflects a need to prove one's bravery to self and others? Which act represents heroism and which heroics? Actually, this question itself is misleading, for the same act can be the action of either a hero or a person engaging in heroics. The key lies within the person, while the realistic value of the act is the same whatever its motivation.

A basic difference between heroism and heroics lies in the degree to which each person has a need to seek out the situation in which a brave act can be performed. Is the woman who rushes into the burning building one who chases fires? The strong person does not necessarily seek out situations in which he can exhibit his strength and courage. When emergencies do arise, when sudden courageous choices have to be made, or when tremendous energy must be summoned and directed decisively, the strong person is able to act. Having confronted and lived with his own fears, he is not overwhelmed by those feelings that accompany the dangerous or demanding situation. Not immobilized or frightened by his own fear, he is able to perform. Secure within, he does not need to continually prove it to himself or others.

Heroism is an act in which you put another's welfare, or your own internalized principles, as a value higher than mere survival. Heroics, or grandstanding, are for personal gain. An American archetypal hero is, of course, Nathan Hale, who regretted he had but one life to give for his country. He stands in contrast to the grandstander like the showoff who sky-dives into the football stadium at half-time and opens his parachute at the last moment, needing (more than just enjoying) the crowd's adulation and reaffirmation of pseudo-valor. The military "hero" may actually be a hostile guy who found a sanctioned outlet for his aggression; however, upon returning to civilian life, he may find it difficult to readjust because there is no outlet for such behavior once his precarious defenses against hostile impulses have been breached. In one case, a decorated Vietnam veteran accepted a "contract" to kill a local dope dealer for $150.

### The Daredevil or Counterphobic Character

The daredevil represents a typical counterphobic reaction. We stand in awe of the courage of the motorcycle stuntman as he turns his cycle down a narrow corridor in the Cow Palace, as he ducks under a low girder at 60 miles an hour, as he streaks into the main arena and up the ramp to jump his machine over more cars than has ever been done before. Yet, after he has succeeded in doing so, he may need to try to leap a chasm. Is this strength or a basic insecurity manifested in the courting of danger? Is it a defiance of feared death or a wish for death? Only analysis of the stuntman himself can answer such questions. The person engaging in heroics is identified by his great need to prove and exhibit his strength. When bravado represents a compulsive showing of strength that belies a basic fear or insecurity, a counterphobic pattern is present.

Self-conscious and noncompulsive compensation for weaknesses does not add up to a counterphobic pattern. The person who recognizes and accepts the fact of a weakness or disability or feared feeling may choose to compensate for the weakness. The Olympian who overcame crippling polio to become a sprinter, the stutterer who became an eloquent speaker, the upper amputee who paints with his toes, all are people who have chosen to confront their real limitations and have been able to master their disabilities. They are aware of their handicaps and choose to master them rather than deny and fear them. The counterphobic patterns are reactions to fear and insecurity and embody a nonacceptance or denial of their existence. Those whose behavior is counterphobic are attempting to negate a part of themselves, while compensators choose a road built on recognition and mastery of their frailty. The latter road is the road of strength, for it includes full self-acceptance and an effort at inner mastery. Alfred Adler pointed out how many remarkable people have underlying handicaps or "organ inferiority" that serve as a challenge to mastery. Blind and deaf Helen Keller comes to mind as a most obvious example.

A Chicano Ph.D. candidate in psychology at a first-rate university described how, in the fourth grade, he had been told he was mentally retarded and had been placed in a special class. He determined then and there to prove he was bright. Asked what would have happened had he not been so labeled, he replied, "I guess I'd have been just another hood in the Mission District." Such obstacles often break, but occasionally make, a person.

### The Achievement Addict

Because of his competence and upward mobility, it is easy to mistake the merely achieving individual for the truly strong one. This is especially likely to be the case in conventional American culture with its emphasis upon success, getting ahead, and material acquisition. Yet the achievement addict's success also represents a form of pseudo-strength, in contrast to the success of the strong person, whose achievements result from both a desire for competence and concern with contributing to social good and cultural advancement. The driven achiever, unlike the previously mentioned examples of pseudo-strength, is not especially concerned with the reactions of other people, but rather with "objective" criteria, with badges of recognition, with status and position *per se*. Because success overrides interpersonal values, he may ride on or over the backs of others. This achiever derives his sense of self-worth and importance from what he does rather than from what he is as a person. Like the individual who is dependent on the approval or affection of others, the achiever is vulnerable. When external reassurances are lost, in his case, through loss of position or attack from colleagues, his self-esteem suffers and depression ensues. Achievement, like "doing good," can be a way of avoiding criticism. At the age of fifty, the pseudo-strong achiever is apt to look out over his lovely suburban home and wonder what it has all been about. His children do not love him for his accomplishments and resent his neglect of them in favor of pursuit of "success." The accomplishments themselves have no intrinsic meaning to him. Our middle-aged man can try to do ever more of the same in an attempt to ward off depression, or he can begin to reorder his life.

## The Stable Person

The stable person, often modestly successful, behaves in conventional ways, but does not necessarily cling to them for defensive purposes. He is not neurotic, just limited. His potential for growth is untapped rather than blocked. Like the gyroscope, he has a capacity to move and adjust, to stabilize in the face of external change. Unlike stronger persons, however, his adaptability tends to be in response to external demands rather than self-generated. He changes if he needs to, not because he wants to. Not seeking challenge, his growth tends to be slow. In being comfortable with himself, he feels no inner necessity for change. The stable character is likely to be the all-American boy or girl, whose development has proceeded smoothly and who has identified successfully with his or her parents and accepted the values, standards, and mores of the community. He is content, likeable, and competent. He is not especially introspective, perceptive, or intuitive, for he has never had to question himself. He does not help change the system because he is a successful product of it. He may make a good surgeon, but he tends to be a poor psychiatrist. He may be a good teacher, but he is not likely to be an innovative researcher or a creative artist. He feels secure because God is in heaven and the president is in the White House (at least he did until 1973). He is what Roy Grinker, Sr., has referred to as the "homoclite," a nice, normal, but dull guy.

The obvious caricature of our stable person is Bob, born in a small Midwestern city to church-going parents, who provided a home of security, affection, and clear-cut expectations. Bob's father coached Little League baseball and was proud of Bob when he became captain of the high school team and president of the senior class. At State College, he met Carol, lead pompon girl. She went on to get her teacher's credentials while he got his master's degree in business administration. They married only after Bob had attained a junior executive position with International Computer Corporation. Even their best friends do not know that Carol was pregnant at the time and that the date for the already planned marriage was moved up a couple of months. Bob has just been elected chairman of the Service Committee of the Rotary Club. His efforts to provide free school lunches to underprivileged children have met with a good deal of success. In keeping with his wish to be a "broad person," Bob has just subscribed to *Psychology Today*. To expand their geographical horizons, Bob and Carol are thinking of purchasing a motor home. Bob would like to have an MG, but realizes that his Pinto station wagon is more practical. He is looked to as a model by a number of members of the Central High School baseball team, for which he serves as a volunteer coach, because of his happiness, success, and personability. There is nothing really wrong with Bob, but Bob has not reached those levels of integration of which he is capable. As Central City changes, he may be hard-pressed to cope with alterations in his comfortable environment. He will adapt, but he will not lead in seeking creative solutions to the new problems. Furthermore his underlying frailty may never be exposed except in times of crisis.

A more familiar historical example would be a successful banker of the 1930s, apparently strong while comfortable in his bastion of power. He was, in fact, a merely stable person. When the bastions crumbled around him, when he was stripped of the illusions of prestige and influence, he committed suicide in his nakedness and shame.

### The Coper

A modern, largely American version of strength, based in large part on contemporary behavioral science's development of ego psychology, is that of coping. The good "coper," the person who is not overwhelmed by the stresses and vicissitudes of life, who adaptively responds to challenges, is thus defined as the strong person. This book utilizes the coping model as an aspect of strength, particularly in regard to the dimension of "outer mastery." Adaptation, change, and growth are intrinsic *but not exclusive* aspects of our conceptualization of psychological strength.

## INTERPERSONAL COMPETENCE

Most of the examples we present obviously contain aspects from all three dimensions of strength but are placed on the dimension that seems to us predominant. Virility, for example, has aspects of both inner and outer mastery, but seems to find its expression predominantly in interpersonal situations.

### Virility as Strength

Closely related to the power model is the virility model, exemplified by the concept of "machismo" in some Latin American cultures. This "strong" man shows his "huevos" (literally "eggs," equivalent of "balls" in English) by his bravado, sexual athleticism, seductiveness, and defense of honor, the latter concept closely related to the Oriental one of "face." Domination of the home by the male, at least ostensibly, with the wife at the service of the husband as his mother had been to him as a boy, characterizes both traditional Mexican and, in another form, Japanese cultures. In Japan, the geisha indulges and pampers as with a child, while inflating his image of manliness. She treats her client like a baby and simultaneously behaves seductively to induce a sense of virility (which she generally does not permit him to demonstrate). In such societies, affectional bonds tend to be male-male, while the female is more a jealously guarded possession. Related, of course, in an extreme form, are traditional Muslim and Arab patterns with women in purdah.

## The Earth Mother

It is noteworthy and obvious that most models of strength in historical and cross-cultural contexts are male-oriented. Yet in subtle forms many cultures view the nurturant, maternal woman as a model of strength. A variety of earth mother and madonna images, even the Soviet "hero-mother," come to mind. At times, the woman who has taken on a man's role is seen as the strong exception—Queen Elizabeth I, Joan of Arc. Although Ben-Gurion referred to Golda Meir as "the only man in my cabinet," her strength is frequently perceived in maternal ways, as illustrated by ubiquitous stories of her having served chicken soup or homemade cookies to her ministers (and Henry Kissinger!). Hopefully, new and broader models of feminine strength are emerging.

## The Tough Guy

The tough guy is apt to be someone who cannot confront the range of his feelings and emotions and has chosen a simple and unsophisticated manner of coping with the multiplicity of data and the complexity of situations in his life. The tough or hard person seeks invulnerability. He does not have the strength to endure real pain, especially of the emotional sort, and thus manages to avoid feeling it. The strong person can empathize with the suffering of others without being overwhelmed by it. He feels bad about human misery, but can still function in the face of it. Often, those who must continually deal with tragedy are systematically taught "toughness." Policemen, probation officers, social workers, and even psychotherapists are warned against becoming "overinvolved." At the opposite extreme, those who resonate so sympathetically with others that they are in the same condition often are ineffective. In trying to comfort a despairing friend, weeping uncontrollably yourself may reflect understanding and caring but may not be of much help. A person cannot truly help if he does not empathetically perceive what the other is feeling. Effective helpers, in many instances, are routinely weeded out by systems that institutionalize impersonality and toughness. A "Marine Corps" personality may be adaptive for combat, but is so for little else.

To illustrate, both of Paul's parents had been Marines. An ex-Marine himself, crew-cut and a "jock," Paul relished his hard-guy image as an investigative officer. His wife was a former policewoman. Only after he accidentally shot his best friend during an episode of drunken showing off did he face the emotional barrenness of his life, his longing for affection, his ever more violent compensatory hypermasculinity. He said, "I had a drill instructor in my head." Following his brief jail sentence, Paul was able to express his needs to his wife, showed more understanding of his children, and saw more clearly the value of those friendships that were sustained during his personal crisis.

### The Stubborn, the Rebellious, and the Defiant

The stubborn person holds back and will not give out or give in. Unlike the rigid person, he may change his own position but no one else can change it for him. Freud himself changed his own theories fundamentally several times, but he tolerated no revisionism in his ranks of followers. (As an unfortunate heritage of Sigmund Freud's stubborn, though under the circumstances of the times understandable, attitude and in the absence of its dynamic but unyielding leader, psychoanalysis has become relatively ossified since Freud's death.) Accommodation, evolution, and even compromise may reflect greater maturity than agonistics.

The habitual rebel seeks change for the sake of change. A strong person may rebel or even lead a rebellion when other channels for change are blocked. But he neither clings to the familiar for security nor demands change that is not constructive or valid in his terms. He does not rationalize a need for change or disruption through slogans. Whenever possible, he seeks to achieve change through the least disruptive means possible, but when he needs to he stands up for his convictions and is willing to accept the consequences. His motivations for change are not hostile defiance or rebelliousness, but are in the service of growth, compassion, and justice. It is easy to be confused about what sort of leadership reflects strength.

Defiance, indeed, is more heroic than compliance, for it often takes more strength to oppose than to give in. Yet an habitually oppositional attitude is as infantile as is a constantly yielding one in the sense that behavior is still externally determined. "If I say yes, you say no; if I say no, you say yes." The symbolic parent is still in power. Authority or demands automatically trigger anti-parental, oppositional behaviors. Classically, defiant attitudes are felt to arise in the first great struggle between the individual and the demands of society, often around the issue of bowel and bladder control. Difficulties of life experienced during the toddler period can result in either compliant or defiant stances. So, often, adult defiance for its own sake is mistakenly seen as strength, erroneously interpreted as a courageous sticking-up for principles, and stubbornness mistaken for perseverance. Defiance in Nazi concentration camps got many killed. The strong knew how to bide time, how to comply temporarily in the service of their own survival.

### The Power Seeker

A need for power, so ubiquitous in the political, corporate, and even academic worlds, may reflect an underlying feeling of helplessness and powerlessness. Those who seek power often have given up obtaining love. They extract from others what they feel will not be freely given. Hitler was concerned with controlling the world, not with being loved by its populace. Power feeds on itself. The powerful person tends to be surrounded by the weak, who give up their freedom to bask in his protection and to gain vicarious satisfaction by identifying with his power. These sycophants reinforce his sense of omnipotence and inability to do wrong. Soon, they too feel they can do no wrong, that the ends justify the means. More and more, the leader hears what he wants to hear. As such, rather than becoming increasingly invulnerable, which is a basic motivation in power-seeking, he becomes more vulnerable because of his ever-increasing remoteness from the consequences of his behavior and loss of touch with reality. National events surrounding the Watergate scandal of the mid-1970s have so clearly confirmed the old adage that "power tends to corrupt, and absolute power corrupts absolutely." The power-seeking person meets his own dependency needs indirectly by keeping others dependent on him.

Thus, if he succeeds in making others need him he can meet his own needs vicariously and also not fear rejection. The protected have only to do what is expected of them, never having to think or make choices, basking in their protector's power. The twenty-year prison inmate, always subject to the power of those in control, loses his ability to choose and take care of himself and often offends again solely to be taken care of again by the powerful, though hated, parent-surrogate, the prison.

The personal histories of the power-seeking and the grandiose often reveal background situations of powerlessness and helplessness and feelings of insignificance rather than backgrounds of mastery and feelings of personal worth. Because such underlying insecurity requires constant reassurance to be overcome, the power-hungry can never rest, are never sated. Even when an election appears obviously "in the bag," manipulations may be engaged in as "insurance," reflecting this underlying insecurity and compulsive drive toward control through coercion.

The prestige obtained through position and through the ability to coerce does not necessarily connote inner strength. The awe or fear inspired by the powerful should not be interpreted as a reaction to personal strength. Those inwardly strong, though often in positions of leadership and power, have no need to throw their weight around and retain their personal worth and dignity even if the trappings of power have been stripped away. A titan of business and communications, about whom books were written, was amazed to find that a few loyal friends stuck by, some famous in their own right, even after his empire had collapsed about him. He spent the remainder of his life as a much gentler, warmer, and more mellow person when he finally believed in his own intrinsic worth.

The quest for power can ultimately lead to paranoia, in which one's own hostile and avaricious impulses are projected onto others. Just as he constantly suspects plots, the paranoiac provokes others to plot against him. Power-seeking is an elusive way to security. It is very hard for those in positions of power, with attendant trappings of pomp and bevies of yes-men, to retain their perspective about their own humanity. Such people often complain of loneliness. Projecting their own ruthlessness, they constantly suspect the motives of others and compile lists of enemies. The well-being of those commanded is easily forgotten in the service of the need to command. The powerful play on the fears of the weak, while the strong person helps the weak become stronger.

## The Manipulator

A subtle form of power-seeking is seen in the manipulators. They are powerful inasmuch as they seem always to get their own way. When one thinks in survival terms, are they the most fit? They may seem to "do well," climbing the ladder of success on the backs of others. They see relationships in terms of what is in it for them and use a variety of techniques from flattery and seduction through cajoling to power plays to obtain their own ends. They even may use pseudo-weakness and feigned helplessness as a means to gain power and control. While they revel in their success at using others, they remain ignorant of the underlying, unconscious forces that compel them so strongly to manipulate. Their charm is in the service of ingratiation, not an expression of friendliness. The accreditation inspector is wined and dined not because of his likeability. A wife's "sick headache" keeps a hard-working husband from attending his business meeting. The manipulator is dishonest. She does not say in so many words, "I resent your spending so many nights away from home"; she controls through deviousness. Is she stronger than her husband?

## The Martyr

The martyr does not want merely to be liked, but to be needed and to have a sense of personal sacrifice. He gives, not out of abundance, but to obligate or even to suffer. He feels he does not deserve to receive if he has not paid a price. The martyr often masquerades under a facade of strength. Like the strong person, he may appear to have much to give. He may be always helpful, willing to aid anyone at any time. No need is so inconvenient that he will not make time to fill it. He encourages people to call upon him for help. He seems always to have a smile, never complaining at the moment about any burden, no matter how great. It is easy to call on him for help because one knows that he will be there. In fact, one almost feels obligated to call, because he would be hurt not to be thought of as always ready to be of service. Yet when his help is sought, the recipient may sometimes feel a vague uneasiness or guilt at using it, concerned about not being as giving as his friend. One never seems to be able to repay the martyr for all the things he has done. The martyr may not be able to make contact with people at a deep level by seeking help himself. He does not share deeply the anxieties, the inconveniences, or problems in his life. Afraid to expose himself to obtain direct contact with others, he seeks their affiliation through inducing obligation. He feels that he has to suffer or to sacrifice in order to earn the love of someone else. "If I suffer, I will be loved." After all, masochism has been defined as the act of loving a sadist—if you suffer, then you get loved. What is sought is not the suffering but the love. The martyr will subtly train others to take advantage of him. He will then use their guilt for always taking from him as a means of controlling, demanding gratitude and sympathy as the price for his services. Others give to him out of guilt for not being as "strong" and giving as he is. They assume the problem is their own inadequacy as givers rather than the result of his subtle manipulation of their attentions.

It is difficult to realize, when in the midst of a complex relationship with this type of person, that serving provides the martyr with the most direct human contact that he can risk. Underneath his helpful facade is a fear of being rejected, low self-worth, and a feeling of having to buy love. The martyr's helpfulness serves to set people up to be sympathetic to his plight. He gives more to receive than to help, though there often is an element of identification with the recipient as one who gets what the giver wishes to receive (but actually may not be able to accept). It is difficult to be angry or to call someone on his martyrdom without feeling guilty at being ungrateful for all the help that the martyr has given.

### The Unenlightened Altruist

The unenlightened altruist gives because he feels that in some sense he "ought to" or because "it is the good thing to do." He gives not because he is full and good, but to try to meet a definition. He may be trying by his "good works" to ensure a place in Heaven. He follows slogans, not his heart. He may avoid guilt, but does he find meaning?

### The Popularity Seeker

The power seeker and the manipulator need to evoke responses in others in order to compensate for lacks within themselves. In a far more benign way, so does the popularity seeker or "love addict." Just as the powerful person is often seen as a model of strength, so is the well-liked person. Likeability is not an indication of true strength in and of itself any more than is the ability to exert power. The strong person is likeable as a by-product of his intrinsic characteristics and of his thoughtfulness, empathy, and concern for others. He does not directly seek to be liked.

Love addicts require the constant reassurance of others' personal regard, even if superficial, to believe themselves worthwhile. The popular individual may not be concerned with the righteousness of his beliefs, only with their acceptance. His concern is with the number of people who like him, less with the depth or quality of the relationships. Courting disparate people, he is likely to run into conflicts of values by attempting to please those whose views of life differ greatly.

### The Hail-Fellow-Well-Met

Closely related to the popularity seeker is Uncle George, a hail-fellow-well-met. He is the most friendly person at a party. He is envied for his ability to establish "instant friendships." George has a smile for everyone and a hearty handshake. There isn't a person he doesn't like. In five minutes of conversation, he can find ties with almost anyone. His brother went to the same college as mine; his mother's neighbor is my little girl's first-grade teacher; his cousin works with my father's brother. His facility in making people feel at home and in involving them in his life through these various connections is a skill to behold. Acquaintances often hold him up as a model or ideal toward which to strive. Because he takes such an interest in others, he is easy to like immediately. Perhaps here is a strong person. He does not seem beset by anxiety about meeting people, nor does he have those petty dislikes for people on first impression. He is outgoing and not afraid of taking the risk of establishing contact with other people. His social skills are obvious. To others, he may seem everything they are not. The trouble is that he is not everything that he seems. Strength means taking the risk of being congruent, taking the risk of being intimate. The hail-fellow-well-met may be very genuine in his friendliness. He may indeed feel the warm feelings that he expresses. Thus, he is not a fraud. However, he is able only to reveal one part of himself, the friendly part, the good half. He does not accept nor share the other parts of his experience: his down side, his anxieties and dislikes. These parts he controls, hides, or represses. Herein lies his weakness: he cannot accept all of himself and share that with others. George is a lonely person, largely untouched by others. He recognizes vaguely his needs for contact and intimacy and tries to meet these needs by increasing his efforts to be friendly. He tries to meet all of his needs for sharing through one mode. His handshake is an expression of anxiety; it is his crying out; it is his depression and need.

### The Fun Lover and the Sensation Seeker

A "flashy" way of life, either in terms of ostentatious materialism or of perpetual high living, often reflects inner emptiness. Insatiable needs to get, rather than to have and cherish, substitute for a deficient internalized sense of worth. Such insatiability is a consequence either of deprivation or, in contrast, of overindulgence, with resultant inability to tolerate frustration. Constant entertainment and amusement can distract from awareness of such emptiness and substitute for absent meaningfulness and positive emotions and relationships. The pretentious and pleasure-seeking are often the jaded, who have succeeded in dulling their experience of life. Lacking intimacy and meaningfulness in life, they require a continuity of new experiences, new highs, new activities. When the novelty wears off, boredom and ennui are common results. This malady is particularly common to the jet-set life style. Sensation seeking and experiencing merely for the sake of the experiences form an identity that is ephemeral and deteriorates rapidly with age. Once it crumbles, there is neither internal strength nor a set of consistent values left to provide guidance and direction to life. The promising but chaotic and drug-filled life of Jean Harlow and other film stars comes to mind.

Though "sowing wild oats" may have a transient usefulness as a phase of adolescence, perpetual and exclusive play in the absence of goal-directed activity and lasting relationships weakens motivation. The glamorous may not be very strong. It is an unhappy commentary on our times that the neurotic, oft-married movie star or the billionaire's wife with her couturier wardrobe, yacht-board parties, and restless unhappiness are seen as ego ideals.

### The Autonomy Worshipper

The strong person cannot be dependent on others for his sense of worth. In that sense, he is autonomous and has a sense of completeness and wholeness. He wants others rather than needs them. The autonomy worshipper or isolate, on the other hand, avoids emotional involvement and reliance upon others. Essentially, he is doing violence to his own humanity in the face of the intrinsic interdependence of man. His position may show more strength than that of the infantile, clinging individual, but still serves defensive purposes. He seeks invulnerability in the face of basic distrust and fears of the unreliability of others. His proof of independence can be a way to deny and ward off wishes to be taken care of. Many sail precariously between the Scylla of feared dependency and engulfment and the Charybdis of feared rejection and isolation, operating within a narrow range of distance from others, moving toward when someone retreats, moving away when someone advances—never meeting. The adult may cling to distance when closeness has not been predictably gratifying, when basic needs have not been met or, in contrast, when closeness has been engulfing, stultifying, or serving the needs of the "giver" rather than meeting those of the recipient (the mother who feeds her child when she herself is hungry). Such distancing, unlike true autonomy, betrays its roots in feared dependency.

Not to be confused with the genuinely autonomous person, who is aware of his needs for interrelatedness, is our autonomy worshipper. George Bach characterizes such a person as accepting "a currently fashionable rationalization of non-intimacy, which in effect holds that one ought not to be much changed or governed by a relationship with another and should just do one's 'own thing.' " A currently widely circulated quotation from Frederick Perls epitomizes this person, who is thus mistakenly identified as strong:

> *I do my thing, and you do your thing.*
> *I am not in this world to live up to your expectations,*
> *And you are not in this world to live up to mine.*
> *You are you and I am I,*
> *And if by chance we find each other, it's beautiful.*
> *If not, it can't be helped.* *

If the autonomous strong person did not make an effort to share himself with others, he would never make contact with anyone. But he can choose involvement. He does not have to leave his life up to chance. He does not watch life happen to him. Taking the risk of being known takes effort and evokes anxiety. In pursuing strength, you must be willing to take this risk, thus being neither an isolate—an autonomy worshipper—nor a clinging vine. A strong person tends to be skilled and autonomous, but knows that he must continue to find and experience himself in interdependence with others.

### The Isolate

One does not have to live in a cave to be an isolate. A person is an isolate when he is afraid of people and does not share himself with others.

The isolate is often the rock that has no feelings, the person who has

* From F. S. Perls, *Gestalt Therapy Verbatim.* © Real People Press 1969. All rights reserved.

no involvement, who knows no hurt. Isolation usually is not chosen because it offers a rich and valuable experience in one's life, as is the case during a spiritual retreat, but more often because of fear of hurt, rejection, loss of control, or being misunderstood. These are all risks that require strength to face voluntarily. In this regard, the isolate is not a strong person. The hermit stands in contrast to the prophet. The hermit loses a sense of himself by withdrawing from interaction with others, while the prophet gains a sense of himself by temporarily withdrawing from others in order to gather his thoughts and strengths.

An isolate may be surrounded by others. He may even serve others. A world-famous neurosurgeon started rounds at 7:00 A.M., rarely left the hospital before 8:00 P.M., and seldom took a vacation. He was contemptuous of those of his trainees and colleagues who were less "dedicated." He rationalized his own emotional impoverishment. His work was a defense, though indeed it served mankind. Dr. X could not love in a personal way. His occupation served to sublimate or indirectly to meet in acceptable ways affectionate, aggressive, and competitive strivings while simultaneously serving the function of emotional isolation.

### The Universal Lover

A contrasting sort of isolate is the person who loves everyone. Mary is "with it." She takes to whatever man she currently dates. She is always around others. She is addicted to encounter group weekends, where she can turn on emotions at will. Instant intimacy with strangers provides few risks. She is concerned about social issues and dedicates herself to liberal causes. Loving everyone, she really loves no one; she is concerned about humanity, not human beings; yet few would be aware of her underlying aloneness. Mary's "lovingness" is in contrast to a feeling of universal love, of oneness and harmony with others that is often experienced most intensely in those times of inner fullness when you are close to realizing the totality of your human potential.

### Autonomy and Aloneness versus Isolation and Loneliness

Although the autonomous person may share some of the characteristics of the isolate, the two are very different. The autonomous person is often highly skilled in the tasks of life, able to function for periods of time without the constant deep involvement or help of others. His needs for love and attention are still real for him, but not as demanding as for many others. Though he wants to relate, he is not driven by an overwhelming need to relate. He is markedly different from the successful, but emotionally isolated, person in that he both can and does *choose* to relate to and share himself with others. He is able to allow himself to be interdependent without fear of losing his ability to cope, his control of himself, or his individuality. Besides having self-awareness, the autonomous person is in touch with his needs for human contact and sharing. He knows that at times we all need the help and comfort of others, that sharing anxieties and troubles increases his affirmation of himself as a whole person. Because he is aware of his ability to function autonomously, he is apt to seek involvement actively, knowing that he becomes more of a person as he shares himself more fully in relationships with others.

It might be construed from this chapter that loneliness is a characteristic of the isolated person but is largely foreign to the strong person. However, as Thomas Wolfe has pointed out,

> . . . loneliness, far from being a rare and curious phenomenon, peculiar to myself and to a few other solitary men, is the central and inevitable fact of human existence.

Clark Moustakas distinguishes between existential loneliness and interpersonal loneliness, saying that every man must face existential loneliness. Interpersonal loneliness, however, can be overcome, depending upon the quality and extent of a person's involvement with others. The isolate must confront both kinds of loneliness. In George Bach's words, "All loners are grappling with the same private dilemma. They are trying to exist psychologically alone and bear the stress of isolation rather than live as authentic twosomes and bear the stress of intimacy."

Existential loneliness is feared by many, driving them into desperate, clinging, dependent relationships in an attempt to escape a feeling that can never go away. Moustakas says, "There is no solution to loneliness but to accept it, face it, live with it and let it be. All it requires is the right to emerge in genuine form." It takes strength and courage to confront your own loneliness and your own fear of being alone openly and honestly. You become a stronger person in your existential loneliness when you use it to grow rather than diminishing yourself by denying your experience. Not only does this help in being in touch with your whole self, but it deepens your capacity for understanding and thus empathizing with others.

The autonomous person does not fear isolation. He does not require others constantly to confirm his sense of existence, as does the child, who gains his very sense of being in the attention he receives from the one initially most important to him—the mother. In this regard, René Descartes' "I think; therefore I am" can be revised to the passive voice: "I am thought about; therefore I am." Charlene was a superb college English professor whose courses were much in demand because of her flair for the dramatic. With her striking beauty and an apparently limitless supply of engaging stories, she seduced both men and women. In the rare case when someone did not respond to her with the attention she needed, she viciously attacked. Above all, she needed to be noticed. She needed to have impact to feel alive and real. She could not be alone.

### The Overly Devoted Person

A newly wedded psychiatric resident refused to remain overnight with his professor and peers during a two-day field trip 200 miles from the university. "We're too close, too much a part of each other, too in love to be apart for even one night." Such incapacity for self-valida-tion can masquerade as love. This clinging ("anaclitic") behavior reflected a lack of boundaries and sense of wholeness. (The marriage lasted less than a year.)

The clinging vine, the person who desperately needs others, often enters into painfully clinging and stifling relationships. To remove the loneliness that is part of every man, he demands of his relationships more than is possible for them to give. He then feels a sense of failure that causes him to search even more desperately for something from his relationships that he can never find. Thus his relationships suffer; people do not want to be around this demanding person, and the weight of interpersonal loneliness is added to the basic existential aloneness that will always be with him. Perceiving the lack of fulfillment of his insatiable demands, he is full of resentment, but cannot express this rage for fear of being further deprived or rejected. His ambivalence is based upon the intrinsic resentment a person in an inferior or weaker position feels toward a stronger person.

## INNER STRENGTH

### The Rigid Person

The rigid person often is mistaken for a person of inner strength, although not so frequently as is the stable person. He is seemingly secure, in touch with and at home with his feelings; he (or she) tends to wear the pants in the family and has enough knowledge to generate a strong personal stand on most issues. He may be a master debater. His opponents come away from an argument with the feeling of not having won an inch of ground, often envious of such strength of conviction and force of character. He always seems to know where he stands on every issue while others debate with themselves and become confused about the complexity of human concerns. Novelty and new information do not fluster the rigid person. Knotty decisions are made easily. He is not confounded by facts. Future shock does not seem to be a problem for him. While others struggle to cope with change and the intricacies of human interactions and agonize over difficult moral and personal choices, he is imperturbable in the face of it all. If confronted with some of the complications of an issue, he often becomes angry with his contenders for their "inability to see things clearly." One often feels inadequate in the face of this "strong" person—for what else could you call someone with unbending moral conviction, someone who stands up for what he believes and who is not afraid to be counted?

When confronted by a rigid person, as we have described him, it is easy to impute inner strength to him, especially if he makes us confront in ourselves areas of ambivalence and indecision. The insecurity that we may then feel often masks from our view his essential weakness—for he, unlike the stable person, is truly weak, as iron is weak in comparison to steel in that it is brittle and unbending. He can allow only limited data and partial aspects of personal experience to be perceived. Any attempt to move him is seen as a threat, hence his frequent outbursts of impatience and anger directed against those who differ from him and impinge upon his unexamined experience. The rigid person is organized along essentially compulsive character structure lines. His need for order and sameness is a defense against inner disorder and uncertainty. Such persons tend also to use obsessive thoughts and ideas as ways of avoiding emotionality and providing certainty.

Firmness and rigidity should not be confused. Were the reader to talk to a person who is rigid and another who is secure, the difference would be recognized immediately. The rigid person tells you that you are wrong, while the firm but secure person shares "where he is at." The person who is both firm and secure in his values, beliefs, and feelings reflects his values in what he does. He tends to demonstrate where he stands rather than to tell you where you ought to be. He comes across as an integrated person. The rigid person, however, is much less comfortable with himself. His words and his actions do not seem to mesh smoothly. His frequent anger and frustration with those different from himself belie his professed security of conviction. A stronger person is able to accept new possibilities, admit new data, and consider alternative viewpoints. He is able to test out possibilities for change in his own experience and then accept or reject them as they have more or less relevance. Being more secure in his sense of himself, he is enabled to incorporate and sample changes in his life without as much fear of being engulfed or invalidated as a person. The rigid person does not have this freedom. To change, for him, would be to deny himself, to say that everything that has gone before is wrong or bad. To change would be to reject himself, to abandon his security; so he clings desperately to a single, unyielding set of beliefs and values in order to protect himself.

The rigid person may appear to be strong, but may fall apart when unable to maintain such patterns through the pressure of circumstances or, on the other hand, when challenges in life or strength of emotions overwhelm this particular type of defense. Basically denying his feelings, when they do emerge strongly, he is not comfortable with them, nor does he have the skills with which to recognize and accept them. He lacks inner mastery, one of the primary requisites of true strength.

Jan was a prominent campus radical. Ostensibly, she defied her father, a retired Air Force general. Her underlying identification with him betrayed itself when, in the heat of emotion at an anti-war rally, she shouted, "Shoot the warmongers!" She was just as uncompromising, dogmatic, authoritarian, and hostile as her father. Whenever confronted with challenge or uncertainty, she waved Mao's little red book, her Bible, exclaiming, "It is all right in here." Fanatics of all political complexions are rigid. Psychological studies have shown similar personality characteristics of those on the far right and on the far left.

Being strong means risking the stress and anxiety of indecision, agonizing over complex moral choices, being willing to seek alternative solutions to problems when existing solutions, though easy to use, are grossly unfair or unsatisfactory.

### The Ultraliberal

By comparison to the rigid person, it might seem that the ultraliberal epitomizes strength. Bill, our hypothetical ultraliberal, has friends from every ethnic group; he proclaims a prejudice against bigotry. He has experienced many different women and a few men. He is experimenting at present with a group marriage and is thinking about joining a commune. He has marched for at least a dozen different causes during the past year—none of which are currently pressing in his life. Valuing freedom and allowing himself to experience anything without fearing engulfment by any particular life style, he has lived with four different people over the past year and looks forward to his freedom to change again in the near future. He has consumed a half-dozen life styles in the past six years and contemplates several more in the next decade. He has been into surfing, drugs, Zen, transcendental meditation, yoga, Rolfing, and is currently taking courses in psychic healing, biofeedback, acupuncture, and hang-gliding. He sees himself and is seen by many others as a person who is uninhibited and free of petty hang-ups about sex, race, and religion—as a person who has been able to transcend the cultural teachings and taboos that stifle most people. He is envied by many in his endless succession of interesting and involving experiences, a truly liberated and strong person. He is, in fact, rigidly flexible.

Before giving the ultraliberal our endorsement as a strong person, let us look a little closer at his qualifications. As a member of the freedom cult, the ultraliberated person is in danger of becoming a sampler in life. The sampler flits from one experience to the next. Always in search of a way to organize and simplify his life, he goes from one philosophy or life style to another and, as the popular song goes: "He is always shopping, never stopping to buy." Because he cannot commit himself to a consistent and abiding set of values, he can never organize his experience in a congruent and consistent way. He will thus be in his person as he is in pursuing experiences: scattered and fragmented. His ability to experience anything and everything without fear of engulfment and without fear of giving up or compromising his identity is founded not in strength but in his knowledge that he has no self to compromise, that he has no commitments to violate. He does have values and beliefs, it is true. Freedom and experiencing themselves are guiding factors in his life. However, these values are often chosen in fear of deep commitment and involvement with any person, idea, or way of life. Without some commitment to a few others who can touch deeply on his experience, who can lend some continuity to his life, who can share both his joys and his frustrations, a person cannot come into full contact with himself.

### The Fanatic

The pseudo-strength of the fanatic can be confused with the genuine strength of the principled person, who sincerely and courageously lives up to his ideals and values. The fanatic rigidly clings to a slogan or creed, which he sees as *the* answer, and which, for him, serves as a security blanket. While the principled person sticks up for what he believes and has a firm sense of the validity of his belief system, he subjects his beliefs to scrutiny, is concerned with their pragmatic implications, and does not impose them on others. His commitments are open to modification by new information. The strong person's sense of identity transcends any one component of his belief system, while the fanatic or rigid person "is" what he believes. To challenge what a fanatic believes is to attack him. The content of the zealot's belief system is not the issue—rather, it is the process by which he holds onto it and attempts to impose it. The totalitarian personality is similar whether the political system he espouses is to the far left or far right. There is a difference between fanaticism and rigidity in the sense that the rigid person may limit himself to defending against any challenge or attack, while the fanatic or zealot attacks others who believe differently. The zealot needs converts to reinforce and affirm his own system. Just as in the political sphere, religious fanaticism takes many forms. Many needs can be subsumed in the guise of righteousness; for example, the free expression of hostile and sadistic impulses in the case of the Inquisition. Ends justify means and genuine principles are lost in the pursuit of an overriding single value. Those who press for "national security" provide a contemporary example of such a rationale.

### Intelligence as Strength

Strength has been assumed by many to lie in intelligence, in wisdom, and talent, which are also seen as having both biological and social evolutionary significance for the human species. Plato's "philosopher-king," the "Renaissance man," and the ancient Chinese reverence for the aged with their accumulated knowledge and experience come to mind. The scientific establishment has enjoyed post–World War II idealization, but disillusionment and frank anti-intellectual sentiment have set in with technology's failure to solve societal problems and its induction of new environmental ones. Cognitive skills are increasingly recognized as worthwhile only in terms of their use in the service of human values and in the context of personal integrity. The deification of science and its achievements has resulted not only in technological monstrosities and ecological disasters but also in intellectual dishonesty in the pursuit of "experimental" results as well as in disparagement of all that is nonquantitative. To accept the limits of the intellect *per se,* to try to place it in personal and social perspective, should not lead to an anti-scientific and anti-intellectual stance, however. The strong eschew simplistic solutions.

### Religious Fervor

Recent popular resurgence of religion and mysticism reminds us that for many, the strongest person is the one with the greatest faith—Job, the Christian thrown to the lions, the Jew dying on the rack of the Inquisition. Another recent Western trend is a burgeoning interest, unfortunately so often superficial, in Eastern thought and practice—Zen, yoga, transcendental meditation, Kung Fu. In such a frame of reference, inner peace and serenity, as exemplified in the countenance of Buddha, in the face of whatever external turmoil, is indicative of strength.

### Pseudo-Identification with a Strong Person

Finally, the most difficult form of pseudo-strength to recognize is that which results from pseudo-identification with a genuinely strong person. The picture presented is accurate, but it is a facsimile, not an original. If strength is a result of mastery and of true identification with a strong person, where qualities of strength have been introjected as part of the self, then actual strength is likely to result. However, observation of a strong person can lead to a pseudo-identification, in which the person only *acts* as if he were strong. He goes through the motions, so to speak, or, in game theory terminology, he plays the game of being strong without actually being strong. Sometimes, this sort of pattern can result from other people's seeing an individual as being strong when he in fact does not see himself in that manner. For example, a child who is big for his age may be seen as strong and mature and is assumed to be the natural leader of the neighborhood kids. He may grow up trying to present a strong and mature image when he, in reality, may not feel this way as a result of his own subjective experience. This person grows up to be the outwardly self-assured executive who is really afraid of people, or the "always loving" person who has been told she is a saint, but who is really hostile and angry inside.

We have exposed the many idols masquerading as models of strength, all of whom bid our allegiance. If we are not to become cynics, we must proceed to the positive avenues through which strength is expressed. Approaching the matter from the inside out, we shall begin with expressions of inner strength.

# 2

# STRENGTH AND MASCULINITY

"If a man could break out of the stereotyped male role, he could put his arms around another man without people thinking he was weird." The comment comes from a 13-year-old boy during a discussion in his "Focus on the Future" class at Union School.*

### Definitions of Masculinity

The concept of masculinity raises many questions. Is the strong man truly masculine? How does one know if he is masculine? Can the unmasculine man be strong? In reality, the questions arising over issues of masculinity and, as we shall see, over femininity as well, are both confusing and complex. Webster's *Third New International Dictionary*, for example, describes "masculine" in several ways:

> having the qualities distinctive of or appropriate to a male; virile, robust, manly; having a mannish appearance, bearing or quality; unwomanly; suggestive of or being in some way like a man; powerful, strong, dominant, forceful, virile, aggressive, vigorous, courageous, forthright.

* *San Jose Mercury-News*, December 10, 1973.

We might turn to characterizations of masculinity in literature, to compound the confusion:

> A man must stand erect, not be kept erect by others. (Antonius Marcus Aurelius)
>
> He is but the counterfeit of a man, who has not the life of a man. (Shakespeare)
>
> The highest manhood resides in disposition, not in mere intellect. (Henry Ward Beecher)
>
> I mean to make myself a man, and if I succeed in that I shall succeed in everything else. (Garfield)
>
> Who dares do all that may become a man, and dares no more, he is a man indeed. (Shakespeare)*

The images reflecting pseudo-strength described in Chapter I make apparent the many ways in which concepts of manliness and strength are intertwined and how various times and cultures have defined masculinity differently. It also is obvious that strength and femininity have usually been defined as incompatible. Not only do cultural definitions of masculinity vary, but most writers seeking to define this basic concept arrive at different descriptions. The guidelines are not clear; the concept is ambiguous. If the definition of masculinity has been problematic historically, the issue is far more difficult in the 1970s in the face of "unisex," the women's liberation movement, and a thrust toward a breakdown of traditional, stereotyped sex roles. Men now serve comfortably as airline stewards and telephone operators, while women recently have served as, or are, prime ministers in Israel, India, and Ceylon. Every man must come to grips with questions revolving around masculinity; the problems associated with this task are numerous. We have consistently noted bewilderment and controversy among our students, more profound in the last few years, when they were asked to discuss the concepts of masculinity and femininity.

I (JAK) remember a time in college when I was especially confused about what it meant to be masculine and anxiously wondered how I was to clarify my confusion. I had entered the office of a professor for an interpretation of the personality inventory we were required to complete in his course. He got right to the point. "Jon, I notice here that you scored high on the femininity scale. I don't think it would be wise for you to consider at this time entering the army." I hadn't even considered going into the service but, faced with the onslaught of a *Doctor* of Psychology and a computer printout, my sense of masculine

* Quotations from *The Dictionary of Thoughts.*

identity was rudely shaken. (Only later did I learn that the scale, in defining "femininity," utilizes items primarily reflecting aesthetic interests, cultural and artistic activities.) In the midst of this confusion, being a little embarrassed and somewhat apprehensive, I approached my college advisor, another psychology professor for whom I had much respect and who had taken a personal interest in me. I remember even now sitting in his living room one evening, finally broaching the subject by asking, "What is masculinity?" "Well," he said, "a lot of men judge their manhood by the length of their penises, but I think that to be masculine is, essentially, to be sure of oneself." I recall being a little puzzled by his comments, for they were not exactly the kind of answer that I had expected. I had hoped for some definitive description of the attributes of, or criteria necessary to rate myself as a man. Knowing these, I expected to be able to relate myself to each of these criteria and then pass self-judgment. Yet I found his words somehow relieving, although I did not fully know why at the time. I did not know that the key to my relief lay in his directing my search from the outside world (with its conceptions of what is masculine) to inside myself (to what I personally valued in my own experience). As is often the case when I reach a personal impasse, I had been searching in the wrong place and asking questions for which there were no clear answers.

## The Semantic Problem

Only later did I understand more fully the wisdom, if not the accuracy, behind the words of my college advisor. Only after reading and comprehending the insights of the general semanticists such as Alfred Korzybiski and S. I. Hayakawa did I more fully come to understand the "tyranny of words" in my own life. "Masculinity" is only a word, a concept, an abstraction. The role of a concept is to point to some reality or to summarize in a shorthand way a set of identifiable data within your experience or in the world about you. Apart from that to which a concept points, it has no independent reality. Yet most of us think of masculinity as being something *real*. You may say, "How absurd. Of course, it is not real," but still most of us "act" as though "masculinity" were indeed real. The concept of masculinity has become reified and perceived as an independent reality. The reason lies in our language itself, which permits us to say: "He *is* masculine." We have this peculiar word "is" in our language (labeled the "is of identity" by the semanticists) that equates people with words. To say that something "is" implies that something exists as a concrete reality. (We are coming to grips further with similar issues in the case of the abstraction "strength.")

What, for example, is the real meaning behind such statements as: "Be a man!" "What *are* you, a man or a mouse?" "You're no man; you're a wimp!" "What kind of a man *are* you?" The implication is that there is something real called a man, which it is possible to "become." Our language thus permits us to say something that cannot happen in reality. Language so colors our outlook on reality and is so taken for granted that we do not often think to question its impact upon us.

So frustrated and angry did I become trying to deal with my own masculinity in this semantic morass that I can still remember coming home from college one day and, taking out my feelings on the typewriter, producing the following chain-of-thought comments about masculinity that expressed the frustration I felt:

a monster

you are a monster, a fiend, you stifle me, i hate you, go away, your existence limits me, your demands warp and confine me, loose me, leave me, i defy you, ah but you are resilient, you are subtle, you sneak up on me in my sleep, my unguarded moments, you haunt me with insidious accusations, you demand a god's wages, worship, reverence, a price i cannot pay, one more soul than i want to give, you do not exist, yet in my denial of you, you gain in stature, oh to deal squarely, to confront, to confine, to define away, to deny, to wish away, but alas you are real in your unreality, i fear i can only win by losing, triumph by quitting the fight, but how to withdraw, i thought that to recognize you for what you are, nothing, a foul creation would be enough, would free me, but i find alas that it is not so, you are not fair, you do not follow the rules, how can I cope, i give, i don't—go away—

he who said that "to create an abstract idea is to create a monster" must have had you in mind, yes, you foul "masculinity"

-jak-

So pervasive is the effect of language on our perception of reality that anthropologists study closely the language structure of a culture in order to have a full understanding of its approach to the nature of reality:

We dissect nature along lines laid down by our native languages. The categories and types that we isolate from the world of phenomena we do not find there because they stare every observer in the face; on the contrary, the world is presented in a kaleidoscopic flux of impression which has to be organized by our minds—and this means largely by the linguistic systems in our minds. We cut nature up, organize it into concepts, and ascribe significances as we do, largely because we are parties to an agreement to organize it in this way—an agreement that holds throughout our speech community and is codified in the patterns of our language. The agreement is, of course, an implicit and unstated one, *but its terms are absolutely obligatory;* we cannot talk at all except by subscribing to the organization and classification of data which the agreement decrees.*

We must remember that a word points to a reality without itself being that reality. Yet most men continue to act, without being aware, as though there were some Platonic ideal of manhood "out there" somewhere, and if we search long enough we may be able to discover it, to incorporate it into ourselves, and at that point to become a man. There is no such "thing" as masculinity, and in thinking that there is we futilely search for what it means to *be* masculine. Yet the concept, like that of strength, still is not without meaning.

### Breaking Stone Tablets

The strategy for discovering the meaning of masculinity and wondering if one "is" masculine is a pursuit doomed to failure if it is a quest undertaken outside one's own experience. The story is attributed to Sören Kierkegaard of the man who was sitting next to the edge of a desert to whom was brought by a parental and wise personage a tablet bearing ten lofty commandments describing the good life: "Thou shalt not kill," "Thou shalt not steal," "Thou shalt not commit adultery," and so on. Here indeed, thought the bearer of the tablet, was the model of how to lead a good and fulfilled life. But the recipient, upon reading the words on the tablet, became infuriated, broke the tablet on a nearby outcropping of rock, and stomped into the desert. There he sat reflectively, looking within, examining himself closely, searching inside himself, recalling his varied experience, seeking his own values and his own conception of "the good life." After many days and nights of painstaking self-examination, he began to chisel his own tablet with great gentleness and care, for this single piece of stone was to contain that which was of central importance to him—a direct expression of his unique experience and perception of the things that were valuable in his life. Completing his tablet, he took it back to show the bearer of the first, now broken, tablet. The man looked at the tablet and read the words: "Thou shalt not kill," "Thou shalt not steal," "Thou shalt not commit adultery," and so on.

* Benjamin Whorf, *Science and Linguistics.*

A more modern and technological version of essentially the same story appeared on television. Atomic war was impending. The great powers agreed upon a moratorium in order that the wisest men of the world in a variety of disciplines might gather together and program a computer with the essence of their knowledge for the purpose of finding out how men could live in peace. Needless to say, the computer printout read: "You should not kill; you should not steal; you should not commit adultery";* and so on. Basic truths must be continually discovered from within oneself, even if one is a computer!

And so it is with "masculinity" (and, as we shall continually emphasize, with *"strength"*). A hundred wise men can come to us with their tablets defining "masculinity"; strength is required to reject these possible "false gods." It requires courage to look inward, having broken the tablets handed us. Being willing to turn inward, being able to relate cultural or societal concepts to your personal experience, is essential. A further step is taken when a person no longer relies solely upon key concepts to define himself, when he can say, "Yes, I *am* a man," "Yes, I am an insurance adjuster," "Yes, I am a father," "Yes, I am married," saying these things to communicate information to another and as aspects of his definition of his own identity, yet wearing these descriptions lightly as a wrap to be shed when not needed or appropriate. Words and concepts are tools to help integrate and understand experience and to communicate with others. They are not to be mistaken for experience itself. You don't discover a sense of identity in vast verbal descriptions of yourself, for, as the aphorism goes, "man defined is man destroyed." Personal uniqueness is far beyond the mere words used to convey yourself to others.

Strength is required for a male to give up the search for masculinity *per se,* to look at his own experience and assess for himself what he enjoys and what integrates his experience. If the behaviors and experiences that you value come close to some of the behaviors culturally described as being masculine, then use the conventional word to describe yourself. However, if what you value in yourself, what you find most fulfilling, what behaviors you prefer to engage in do not approximate the behaviors pointed to by that concept, then it requires courage to say that you are not, then, "masculine." A strong man, rather than seeking to *become* masculine, which is to seek to become something outside himself, is more apt to look at his own experience, the richness and color and texture within it, and out of these raw materials create the kind of person he chooses to be. Each

* From *The Answer,* by Leonard Freeman.

person works with different materials—height, weight, bodily configuration, skills, aptitudes, talents, etc.—so that every person's creation must of necessity be different. To copy another person's creation (to try to become someone else's conception of masculinity) is to deny yourself. When my advisor told me that "masculinity" was being sure of oneself, I was given all the information that I could use at that moment. And I was helped by this nondefinition to begin to turn away from the tablets of others and to turn inward in order to discover myself and my unique values and modes of expression.

### The Freudian Bias

To Freud, who was influenced strongly by cultural norms and who had great impact on defining and reinforcing such norms, anatomy was destiny. Impressed by the anatomical representations in vestigial form of organs of the opposite sex (such as the appendix testis in the male and the clitoris in the female) and later reinforced by knowledge that each sex has some hormones of both, Freud and his followers postulated constitutional bisexuality on the psychosexual level. For Freud, activity as opposed to passivity was the earliest behavioral manifestation of sexual differentiation. An individual responded to external influences on the basis of these inherited trends. A homosexual developmental phase followed the autoerotic and anteceded the heterosexual or genital phase. Oral or anal fixations could predispose toward failure of heterosexual development. As the child discovered the difference between male and female genitals, he or she came to understand the difference between masculine and feminine. The female was initially perceived by the child as a castrated male; femininity involved an acceptance of a penisless, essentially deprived state. Anxieties about a boy's strivings and competition with father for mother could lead to fear of castration, which in turn might result in repudiation of masculine sexual aims and objects. Issues of dependency, aggression, power, and identification readily could become fused with sexual motivations.

Freud consistently underestimated the importance of social factors. As pointed out by a number of female psychoanalysts, his psychology of women was relatively weak, not taking into account positive biological forces of generativity and maternalism. Those having a stake in the traditional sex role system often point to early Freudian conceptualizations to bolster their positions, overlooking more recent psychoanalytic insights. (And those not satisfied with Freud may go back to the Scriptures to bolster their ideas of male superiority.)

### Biological Factors

Sexual difference in behavior among mammalian species are prominent and varied. The male generally is the more aggressive, involved in tests for dominance and in the protection of the group in the social species. However, males of a number of species participate in protection and rearing of the young. Females can be highly aggressive, particularly when defending their offspring, but also when competing for dominance. Sexually specific behavioral repertoires can be modified significantly by castration and by the administration of contrasexual hormones. The steer is far tamer than the bull. Recent research places importance on the hormonal environment during gestation. There is some evidence that, at least for rodents, exposure to high levels of hormones of the opposite sex *in utero* may modify adult sexual behavior, presumably on the basis of neural organization. There is recent suggestive evidence that boys born of diabetic mothers who received high doses of female hormone during pregnancy are less aggressive than those of untreated diabetic mothers. On the other hand, animals of both sexes have the potential for and occasionally exhibit behavior characteristics of the opposite sex. In the male, aggressive and sexual behaviors are closely linked, while in the female, sexual behaviors are closely related to submissive postures that serve to stay the attack of an aggressor. Animal studies, however, do not fully support the notion of the critical difference in general behavior between the sexes as related specifically to activity versus passivity. Even in sexual activity *per se*, the female may be very active.

Other support for the notion of intrinsic biologically based behavioral differences between the sexes comes from the observation of newborn infants in which claims have been made for a preponderance of active exploratory behaviors in the male. (However, major individual differences exist in neonatal behavior within each sex.) It is extremely difficult, however, to separate biological from environmental factors, which come into play very early. The baby boy is given a blue blanket; a pink ribbon is placed on the nearly bald head of the newborn girl, and the family comments, "Isn't she feminine?"

Richard Greene points out that there are three separable and independently determined issues in gender identity: sex of preferred sexual partner, self-concept in terms of social role, and self-concept in terms of anatomical sex. For example, he finds that many adult male transsexuals (anatomically normal males seeking sex-change surgery) were treated like little girls during the first three years of life. Further evidence for the enormous importance of gender assignment for gender identity comes from the case of pseudohermaphrodites, children born with the external genitalia of one sex but the genetic disposition and internal genitalia of the opposite sex. By the age of three, the individual sees himself firmly as a member of the sex in which he or she has been reared. Evidence from cases of genetic error with extra X (female) or Y (male) chromosomes is confusing, because such defects generally occur in conjunction with other disorders such as mental retardation and abnormalities in stature and secondary sex characteristics.

In sum, there is substantial evidence for at least a predisposition to particular behavior patterns depending upon genetic, anatomical, and endocrinological sexual differences. In the human being, how such propensities are developed and modified depends enormously upon the vagaries of psychosocial influences. Whatever the intrinsic differences, the issue is certainly not one of superiority or inferiority. Moreover, social evolution has proceeded at a vastly greater rate than biological evolution. Sex-specific behaviors that are adaptive for the lion or chimpanzee or were so for the caveman, however biologically based, may be maladaptive in contemporary society.

### The Athlete and the Poet

Not grasping fully the true nature of a concept and its relationship to human experience, a person may still ask, "But what about the poet, for example? Is he not less masculine than the athlete?" If he seriously wants to find an answer to such a question, he must first have a firm definition of "masculinity." The answer to his question would be Yes if he defines the masculine man by the following characteristics: (1) he plays team sports—he is a "jock"; (2) he hates ballet; (3) he combs his hair using the "dry look"; (4) his chest is hard and hairy; (5) he has a penis over $4\frac{1}{2}$ inches long in the flaccid state; (6) he is generally assertive to aggressive; (7) he is able to ball seven out of ten chicks by the third date (he also smokes Marlboros, not Virginia Slims!). Having a clear (even if biased) idea of what characterizes masculinity, one can bring forth the poet and the athlete, compare them in the light of the definition, and tell whether or not they meet one's own standards of masculinity. Using the above definition, which is somewhat descriptive of the varied and vague notions people have about masculinity, either the poet or the athlete may qualify, although the athlete is, in our culture, more apt to fit the definition. If the poet does not have time for sports, if he prefers not to be aggressive, if he is not even interested in trying to make it with more than one girl, then he is not appropriately defined, relative to the above characteristics, as being masculine.

The fact that the poet does not meet the criteria of the above list does not really seem very important. It would not make much difference, if it were not for the fact that such high value is placed on this thing we conventionally call masculinity. It is commonly thought and deeply felt that masculinity is good. Masculinity implies strength. A male person who is not masculine is to be looked upon with contempt or, at best, pity. Vague feelings arise that he might be "queer" or weird, or perhaps wimpy, if he is not masculine. Some eighth-grade boys were assigned to go home and say they wanted to become nurses or dental assistants. One boy reported his brother's reaction, "Do your thing . . . but stay away from me!" Another said, "My mother told me I'd become a fag if I was a dental assistant." Where does role and occupational identity end and gender identity begin? In most men, feelings regarding masculinity are unexamined and mixed with high emotion and little clear thought, compounded by the deceptions introduced by our language. When it is said that it is better to be masculine than something else, or that it is better to be a jock than a bard, this judgment is made in the light of some unspoken value. Because of our interest in the psychology of the strong person, let us judge the athlete and the poet in relationship to the values that we cluster with strength.

Does our athlete (also being characterized here as masculine) have a firm sense of himself? Does he acknowledge his needs for interrelatedness, for touching, for helping and being helped? Does he know and care about his teammates, or do they just play games together? Is he capable of gentleness? Is he self-aware and resilient when he encounters stress? Does he have a high degree of mastery over both his inner and outer environment? Does he have the courage to share himself wholly with those few persons to whom he chooses to be close, to acknowledge his fears and weaknesses in addition to his love and affection? If our athlete pursues behaviors culturally defined as masculine out of congruence with his own inner nature and possesses the attributes of strength, we could well say, "Yes, this masculine person is also strong." More often, however, masculine pursuits are followed as a means of proving self-worth and exhibiting external mastery rather than being expressions resulting from self-searching. When this is the case, then this person, thought masculine, may not be best characterized as strong. Thus, although the athlete is held out to most of us as being the epitome of masculinity, he is not necessarily strong. Even more confusing is the athlete who is also overtly homosexual. If so, is he still masculine?

If the athlete is not necessarily a strong person, does this imply that the poet is more closely aligned with the characteristics of the strong person? A question of this sort is best answered relative to our understanding of strength. Again, of a particular poet, we must ask the same questions we did of the athlete. Did he choose to become a poet out of an inner search for his unique path in life? Having qualified on similar grounds, then he might well be described as a strong person.

It is possible, however, that the poet chose his path because he needed to escape his own inner turmoil through aesthetic pursuits, or because he felt himself a failure in competing with others for masculine honors, or as a way of rebelling against his father who wanted him to become a physician and join the ranks of the professionals. Perhaps he wrote of love out of fear of seeking it in life. These would be acts not in response to himself and his own needs and potentials, but in response to inner defenses and outer influences. But if his poetry expresses and creatively handles conflict—if the poet (or artist) dips into his unconscious out of courage and in pursuit of creative solutions, this very act may reflect strength. If, on the other hand, he needs again and again to reassure himself with his words or pictures, his creation, however beautiful, his works become a personal crutch. Creativity can be but is not necessarily a strong alternative to psychopathology. Both tend to arise from conflict, from idiosyncratic experience. We all know that creativity and crippling psychopathology often co-exist, yet the strong certainly may be among the most creative out of their knowledge of themselves and their courage to be different.

In general, a true poet has some advantages in developing strength. In choosing an artistic pursuit, he would not be taking the well-worn path. Many would ridicule and think him effeminate. To feel secure, he must choose this path with firm knowledge that poetry is a congruent expression of himself. Additionally, aesthetic pursuits require a person to be more finely in touch with his inner being. In a culture that makes it difficult to be expressive of feelings, that is preoccupied with development of mastery over the environment, the poet may have a head start over the athlete in terms of knowing and cultivating his inner being. It might be said that the person pursuing masculine activities is more apt to seek external mastery and the artist is predisposed to have greater inner skills. Strength is found in those persons, athletes or poets, who successfully integrate both.

### The Don Juan Fantasy

A special case in one subcult of the masculine ideal is the Don Juan. It takes considerable skill, poise, and self-assurance to be a good Don Juan. His highly developed skill in life is getting women into bed. He has explored the terrain many times. He knows the battleground and knows a multitude of effective strategies. He is a perceptive person, sensitive to the avenues to be followed in bringing his little drama to a climax. Within this arena, because he is so highly knowledgeable, he can be poised and self-assured. Psychodynamically, the Don Juan is highly ambivalent about relating to women. His own development is likely to have been characterized by a period of intense attachment to his mother, followed by a perceived rejection. He attempts continually to recapture a feeling of closeness with a woman in the face of basic distrust. He pays women back by ultimately rejecting them. His only real friends, if he has any, are men.

The thought of being a Don Juan is a powerful fantasy. Just as the playboy fantasy leads many men to imitate the life style associated with this image, so do many consider the life style of the Don Juan to be the height of both masculinity and the good life. And for many women, tired of trying to relate to dull men who are afraid to risk sharing themselves, the poise and confidence of the Don Juan is appealing. The excitement associated with his direct appeal to the often untouched sensuality of a woman frequently makes him very attractive to her. He helps confirm her adequacy as a sexual person. Women, too, need to be touched and held. On an unconscious level, he often plays into the masochistic needs of some women to be hurt, to see men as rejecting or unfaithful. The chance to meet these needs in relationship to the confidence and seeming masculinity of the Don Juan may make him irresistible.

If a person has to choose between being an average person, going through life neither sharing much of himself nor being touched deeply by others, and being a Don Juan, not relating deeply, but having exciting and titillating adventures with a variety of women, it would be hard to say why the latter might not be the preferable course. The Don Juan has a considerable degree of external mastery. But when compared to a strong person, he lacks the inner mastery and self-awareness that characterize the strong person. He never really finds love, but forever seeks it. This pattern may not be immediately noticeable, however, for today he probably has more sophistication even in his internal awareness than in the past. It is not uncommon to find many a modern Don Juan, a product of the encounter generation, coming across to women with genuineness and honesty of sorts. The use of honesty as a "line" is one of the many strategies that the competent Don Juan has in his repertoire. In fact, he has undoubtedly "bagged more than one trick" with the use of pseudo-honesty and genuineness. It takes careful self-discernment even for the strong person to differentiate between using his ostensible congruence and honesty strictly to achieve some end—e.g., sex—and genuinely attempting to present a transparent congruent expression of himself.

There are some Don Juans who eventually do discover, as one day they are overcome with loneliness and depression, the reality of their impoverished existence. The swinging singles apartment complex has been the brainchild of more than one developer who has sought to capitalize on the fantasy many people entertain of living the playboy experience. One married man's single friend, who rented a luxurious singles-only apartment, was envied, for he was about to fulfill the fantasy common to almost every man—beautiful women, nonstop parties, unlimited opportunity for unencumbered sex. At the time of this writing, an initially full local complex is advertising for couples and marrieds to fill its many empty apartments. Parties became dull, the continual demand and expectation for sex became less interesting, and playing musical rooms disorienting. The strutting, primping, and other mating-game displays around the pool became a distraction for those who wanted to swim. Forced to live the carefree, *Playboy* magazine-type existence, many renters found the life unfulfilling and lonely. The idea was to share in the fun, to share one's body, to enjoy. But who was there to share the times of loneliness, frustration, depression, and conflict? As large areas of their experience were continually untouched, the residents became more and more alone and unshared. Many left, searching for other values, other fantasies to pursue, and other paths to follow. But for these, a service was done. So many people harbor consistent fantasies about super-masculinity and the playboy life, that everyday existence pales by comparison. Nothing done in the routine of life can measure up to the exciting promise of the fantasy; in comparison, daily life is perceived as a bore. Many spend a lifetime resenting and finding dull the "average" persons around them, always imagining the exciting life that could have been open to them if it were not for being married, tied down, or otherwise prevented from pursuing their dream. Feeling this, they never consider that, if given a chance to live their fantasy, it might be found lacking.

### *Following in Others' Footsteps*

I (JAK) am, in my own life, reminded of this truth time and time again as I find myself trying to follow someone else's path, trying to become some image of how I would like to be that is different from how I am at a given moment. Traveling in Europe for the first time (not alone), I had my knapsack full of guides, including Frommer's *Europe on $5 a Day*. I visited all the famous museums, went to the sidewalk cafes, sat many long hours over coffee and croissants, tea and crumpets, beer and pretzels, or wine and cheese, and talking intently with fellow travelers I chanced to meet. I saw a dozen countries and I felt awful. Here I was doing what my friends fantasied doing. How could I not enjoy myself? How could I not find each second exciting and interesting? Everyone I met seemed to be able to do this. Why couldn't I? I pulled myself aside to meditate a bit on why I was feeling so depressed. In doing that, I rediscovered a truth that I had previously known and forgotten: I was following someone else's footsteps, trying to be interested and to enjoy every minute. In reality, I was ill-prepared to travel in countries in which I did not know the language. The constant hassle just of getting from one place to another logistically, trying to be understood, finding a place to sleep, and deciding where to go next was very stressful and, at times, upsetting. I was not sharing or acknowledging this part of my experience. I discovered that my preference, when I thought about it carefully, was to go to one place and try to become a part of it for a time—not to flit from place to place and person to person. I almost felt guilty for not wanting to see everything that I "should." So I began to share with others whom I met the anxieties that I felt, asking them how they coped with constant change and what was their conception of how best to travel. I went to a small island off the coast of Spain, became part of a small community, and stayed for a while. I felt better, for I was finally charting my own path rather than following that of someone else.

The Don Juan and the playboy life style are travel guides introduced by someone else. They represent a way of living and, most likely, defenses that do not necessarily have relevance. If you try to become what a Don Juan represents for someone else, you deny yourself—you may feel lonely, unshared, and probably eventually anxious and depressed.

### The Either-Or Trap

A second characteristic of man's thinking, in addition to the "is of identity" of language, is the either-or form of reasoning so tied up with Aristotelian logic. Things tend to be perceived as being either good or bad, true or false. We are told to make up our minds—yes or no—like a binary digital computer. This on-or-off kind of thinking is subtly pervasive throughout our daily transactions and is at the core of a common problem of many men seeking to assess their own masculinity. As pointed out, masculinity is often equated with strength, particularly with simplistic concepts of strength in terms of achievement and prowess. Moreover, as indicated by Lionel Ovesey, our culture places a premium on self-assertion, and the man who lacks it and fails to meet success goals is plagued with doubts about his masculinity. Thus, any adaptive failure—sexual, social, or vocational —may be perceived unconsciously, as a failure in the masculine role. Furthermore, symbolic extension through the equation says I am a failure = I am castrated = I am not a man = I am a woman = I am a homosexual leads to intensification of the original anxiety.

No man can avoid asking himself or being asked by others in some form or another the question, "Are you a man?" Our culture does not have a clear rite of passage from adolescence to manhood; nor, as we have seen, does it provide a clear definition of masculinity with which to gauge progress, yet it is clearly held out as an ideal to which every man "ought" to strive. How do you know the day when you change from being a child, or adolescent, or juvenile, or youngster to being a man? What magical thing makes the difference; what clearly has to change? Is it when you graduate from high school, when you turn 21 (or is it 18 now?), after you have "made it" with your first chick, after you get loaded for the first time, after you finally beat someone up, after you leave home for good, when you start smoking a pipe, or when you can ski down the face? When? How?

With all of these competing answers to the question, it is very difficult for you personally to know when you are a man. And, consistent with our either-or logic, you may be asked, "Well, are you a man or aren't you?" No doubt is permitted. To be unsure is considered unmanly. Yet, how are you to know in the face of the ambiguity of the question? Doubt is the rule rather than the exception in our culture. And it is at this point that many men have problems, in part semantically based, with the question of their own masculinity. Not being able to answer with total assurance that they have finally passed the proper test of manhood, they make the assumption in either-or fashion that "if I am not masculine, or if I even doubt my masculinity, then I must be effeminate. If I am effeminate, I must be homosexual." Actually, effeminacy is a caricature rather than an accurate representation of feminine traits based on a variety of neurotic defenses, including hostility toward and ridicule of women. It is surely possible to have feminine traits without being effeminate. Moreover, so-called masculine and feminine traits are not mutually exclusive. Receptivity, intuitiveness, and aesthetic sensibility are compatible with such things as assertiveness and interest in sports.

It is not at all uncommon for men-boys in the long transition between adolescence and manhood to jump from questioning their masculinity to being concerned about being gay. Thousands of men, finally getting the courage even to talk about it, come to counseling centers on college campuses for this reason. The following kinds of comments are predictable among them: "I haven't been able to make it with a girl. Does that mean that I am a homosexual?" "I prefer being around men rather than women—I must be gay." "I really enjoy cooking and knitting. I wonder if that means I am gay—I guess I would make some man a good wife." Any sense of failure or weakness or awareness of passivity may lead to fear of homosexuality, even in the absence of any actual libidinal attraction to men. In addition, wishes or strivings for a dependent relationship with a powerful man may lead to such fear (and, of course, may at times be a component of overt homosexuality). Dependency and power issues prominent in neurotic forms of homosexual relationships are certainly not absent in conflictive heterosexual relationships as well. Aside from the concern about "feminine interests," meeting a gay first-string defensive tackle may also precipitate anxieties about homosexuality; it may not be possible merely to write him off as a "nellie fag," clearly different from yourself.

### The Role of Parents

The problems associated with becoming a man are inherent in our culture itself. The extent of the problem in a given boy's becoming a man is determined in large part by the nature of his interaction with his parents and other significant adult figures in his life. If his relationships to these important adult models are good ones, then the problems posed by our culture and language will be minimized. Obviously, the father plays a crucial role. In trying to sort out the influence of parents on their male child, it helps to think of one parent (the father) providing the son with a model that strongly influences his self-concept and the other parent (the mother) providing the child with his first relationship with a woman, the success of which helps determine his later choice of a sexual partner. The mother also can either foster or impede the relationship with father. The mother-father relationship itself serves as a model for man-woman relationships for both the boy and the girl.

A healthy boy who is predisposed to heterosexuality is most likely to have had a warm father who was sure of himself and his own masculinity and with whom the son could positively identify. This process provides the son with the major foundations of his own self-concept. If his mother was nurturing, unrejecting, and warmly involved with her son and allowed his gradual identification with and emotional involvement with his father, then the son will be strongly inclined, when he becomes more independent of the family, to seek support, affection, and sexual gratification from women, whom he then sees as loving and trustworthy, and of whom he is unafraid. Thus, a child typically derives his self-concept from the same-sex parent and is largely influenced in the sex of his object-choice or sexual partner by the parent of the opposite sex. "I want a girl just like the girl who married dear old Dad," goes the song.

A man who had a good relationship with his mother, predisposing him to later good relationships with women, but had a fouled-up relationship with an inadequate, rejecting, or cruel father tends to feel confused about his own identity and to be unsure of himself as a man. It is unfortunate that in our culture, with much blind faith in and misconceptions of masculinity, many a father avoids giving warmth and affection to his son. The fear is that if he were to do such things as putting his arms around his son, hugging him too much, holding his hand, or having any form of affectional contact with him he will encourage his son to later homosexuality. Thus many fathers remain emotionally aloof and, in the process, make it difficult for the son to have a firm sense of self through close identification with the father. Then, when the son is later faced with sexual choices, he will have less basis on which to feel adequate and sure of himself as a man. Homosexuality itself may result not only from hostility toward or fear of women, but from the seeking of love from a man because it had not been given by the father in childhood, or from the human attempt to introject (take in) the masculinity of the sexual partner in the face of failure or identification with the father.

Frigidity in a man, either in the form of emotional coldness toward women or in the form of impotence or premature ejaculations, usually has its roots in the man's initial relationship with his mother. If the primary experience a man has relating to a woman is with his mother for ten, fifteen, twenty years or even longer in these days of extended dependence on the primary family, and if he is fearful or aversive on the basis of either rejection or engulfment, then he is not going to have had much practice relating emotionally and intimately or in a good way with a woman. Fearing closeness to a person of the opposite sex, it is understandable why he would then prefer to keep an emotional distance from a woman in order to protect himself, thus sowing the seeds of frigidity. His premature ejaculation may be a way of denying the unconsciously hated woman her pleasure. It will take either psychotherapy or an unusually understanding and nonthreatening woman to overcome this man's initial fear and anxiety related to the primary woman in his life.

Similarly, in a culture that devalues women, which ours has done to a considerable extent, it is difficult for some husbands to love their wives. To love one who is not esteemed is difficult. It is difficult to love an unequal. To the extent to which a mother is devalued in a culture, the ability of a man to relate meaningfully and intimately with a woman is reduced. An extreme example of this situation was the ancient Greek culture, in which women were of very low worth and the primary emotional relationships were among men and homosexuality abounded.

In our own culture, men in certain "womanly" occupations are looked upon by other men with disdain as being feminine. In America, for example, male ballet dancers have been considered to be in a feminine occupation; whereas, in the Soviet Union, it is considered a masculine pursuit. Apparently, gay men are more frequent in American ballet than in Russian. Straight American male dancers are forced to make a point of their heterosexuality, as are straight hairdressers. Those with heterosexual inclinations are systematically discouraged from childhood from occupations for which they may have talent and interest. In contrast, the woman with aspirations for a "masculine" occupation such as medicine or engineering, perhaps respected in a way for having to overcome prejudice, is often considered to be "coming up in the world."

A man might have had a good relationship with his father, providing him with a good self-concept, but may have been rejected and put down by his mother. Not having had much emotional closeness as a child from a woman, he may later turn to men in homosexual relationships as his choice of sexual partner. His object choice of men may occur even though he still has a firm sense of himself as a man, derived from a good relationship with his father.

Such homosexuals tend to be "masculine" in manner and may prefer the "active" (inserter) sexual role. It should be clear that there should be both a significant male adult with whom to identify and from whom to derive a sense of self and a significant woman from whom to derive emotional support and affection for facilitation of a boy's ease of eventually entering into heterosexual relationships.

Apart from the broader issues involved in the respective and appropriate roles of men and women and their legitimacy, it is currently confusing in our culture for a child to have parents who have reversed roles. If a boy has a passive, unassertive father and an assertive to aggressive mother, he may have problems, even if the parents are comfortable with their own roles and relationships, in that he will come up against societal definitions vastly different from his familial ones.

### The Son of a Unisex Couple

An interesting situation of current vintage has resulted from the unisex movement, in which both parents may dress similarly, wear long hair, and divide the household roles equally or according to convenience and talent rather than based on traditional conceptions of what is appropriate masculine and feminine behavior. The intriguing question immediately pops into mind: Is this a breeding ground for sexual confusion and deviancy? Who hasn't heard the comment about a couple in the street: "Which one is the girl?" or had the somewhat confusing experience of being initially attracted by someone mistakenly taken for the opposite sex?

Surprisingly, many aspects of unisex couples may be quite conducive to fostering self-confident heterosexual men. Many of the men partaking of the unisex look have a firm enough sense of self to be willing to appear different. In addition, they have typically rejected some of the more destructive components of the cultural image of masculinity, i.e., the need to be aloof and self-contained, not to cry, to be tough. Freed of some of these kinds of constraints, they often relate to their own sons in a much more emotionally and personally involved way, thus providing the son with a firm sense of himself and much more comfort with his own feeling self than is possible with cold and aloof fathers. The women who are self-confident enough to break from the cultural mold and are willing to relate to other than a super-masculine, controlled, unemotional male are often themselves more self-confident as persons. Too, they are more likely to value the human and feeling qualities in men. Valuing these qualities, they are apt to relate well on a feeling level with their sons, thus providing them with a firm foundation for later relationships with other women.

This is not to give a blanket endorsement to the couple with completely undifferentiated sex roles. Many people choose this pattern not as an authentic expression of firmly held personal values, but rather out of rebelliousness against their own parents and other parental figures around them, out of the need for identification with a subgroup in order to gain a sense of identity, or because of anxiety about the opposite sex which then must be "disguised." But the virtues possible in this movement should not be overlooked out of prejudice, either. Certainly, a unisex couple can produce, and may even have some advantage in producing, well-rounded and healthy children who ultimately may help move society in more wholesome, less constricting directions.

### The Masculine Homosexual

Of the young men who do leave their homes with a predisposition for homosexuality and who encounter life circumstances that introduce them into the gay world, the questions of masculinity are not necessarily resolved in choosing the gay path. Many homosexuals in gay bars prefer masculine-appearing men, well developed and muscled. The idea is often implied: "If I can screw a masculine man, then I feel that I am more masculine than he is." The motive of many men for homosexual relationships is not a striving to become more feminine, but rather a seeking for being close to and accepted by other masculine figures, thus confirming and enhancing their own shaky sense of masculinity. The queen (a female-posing homosexual) is, therefore, in poor demand on the streets, but finds a much larger market for his form of homosexuality in prisons. The men in prisons often turn to homosexual relationships not out of a basic predisposition to this form of behavior, but because no other form of outlet is available. These men seek the closest thing to a woman they can. Thus, the feminine homosexual is more attractive to them than a masculine-appearing one would be.

### Motorcycles and Leather

Another current phenomenon is the leather bar, typically associated with the motorcycle set. Here, the expressions of manliness are actual charades of masculine behavior, "butch drag." Strong fetishistic, as well as sadomasochistic, elements appear. Super-toughness, super-coolness, swearing, fighting, aggressiveness, boisterousness, and other exaggerated forms of masculine behavior are the rule. Having had hostile and distant relationships with their fathers or other primary male parental figures, these men both express through sexual behavior and deny through hypermasculine behavior feminine wishes, while simultaneously being "tougher" than the feared father. Within a homosexual relationship, many a very masculine-appearing male will assume a passive role. Many men, not being able, in a traditional masculine context, to integrate dependency needs, needs for gentleness, needs to be taken care of, needs sometimes to be passive instead of always assertive, find within the passive role a way of meeting these needs. We do not mean to suggest, however, that the choice of a gay or bisexual life style implies for the man either lack of strength or of masculinity. It may have authenticity and certainly can require courage.

The problems of definition and pursuit of masculinity are many and inescapable. They exist for every man and are generally difficult to resolve clearly. The resolution of the masculinity crisis is fraught with emotionality and subtle semantic and cultural traps. It is a wonder that as many men come to a firm sense of themselves as actually do. We have not succeeded in finding a definition for masculinity in the semantic sense, nor have we really tried, for every man grows in strength by finding his own.

# 3

# STRENGTH
# AND FEMININITY

Just as the strong man has problems in becoming fully human in the face of stereotyped social roles defining masculinity in terms of prowess, achievement, and toughness, so, too, does the strong woman face major challenges in integrating competence and equality with a unique sexual identity. Obviously, there is no simple way to define femininity, an abstraction as elusive as masculinity. Moreover, femininity, female roles, and the concept of the strong woman are currently issues of controversy and flux in the face of the so-called women's liberation movement, out of which hopefully will arise new models, a broader range of choices, and new freedoms rather than merely new cultural stereotypes.

## The Dearth of Models

We have presented strength as encompassing inner, interpersonal, and outer dimensions, arising from senses of inner peace and personal identity, from the capacity for intimacy, and from outer capability

This chapter was written with the assistance of Pat Howe and Diana Bunce, many of whose views are reflected, along with the authors', throughout the chapter.

and competence. As discussed previously, men are often handicapped because they are exposed to many models of outer strength, accomplishment, achievement, power, and ability. Often arriving at a sense of identity and masculinity from their fathers, men frequently perceive themselves as men because they are able to do things, to be successful. In doing thus, they often neglect inner development, the ability to be vulnerable, the ability to share weakness, the ability to recognize and handle feelings. Lack of feeling awareness is a major problem characteristic of men in our culture. There is a dearth of male models for this aspect of strength.

For women, the problem is the reciprocal. In our culture, they are much more apt to be reared to be more responsive to their feelings, but not given models of feminine accomplishment and competence outside the home. This is not to say that a housewife is not competent at many tasks, but it is to say that, in terms of a career or vocation, there are few women to act as inspiration or as guideposts for those who seek other kinds of achievement. For most women, there are few women emotionally close enough to fulfill this competent ego-ideal (model) function. Moreover, women of achievement may seem incomplete in terms of their noninstrumental ("typically feminine") roles.

### Emulating Men

Some women, faced with this lack of models, yet still attempting to enter into what has been described as the "man's world," have tried to emulate males, becoming one of the boys and, in the process, forsaking feelings, awareness, and responsiveness. The aggressive, boisterous, drinking, swearing woman executive epitomizes this person. She is a female version of the male chauvinist pig the feminist is supposed to despise. She has not only taken on a male model, but an archaic one at that. On the other hand, the relative lack of feminine models of worldly achievement permits the creative, strong woman a greater latitude in defining herself, in achieving a unique identity free from cultural stereotypes.

### Integrating Masculine Values

A recent statement of the Boston Women's Health Book Collective comes to grips with issues of old and new stereotypes. "We all went through a time when we rejected our old selves and took on the new qualities exclusively. . . . But ultimately we came to realize that rejecting our 'feminine' qualities was simply another way of going along with our culture's sexist values. . . . In no way do we want to become men; we are women and proud of being women. What we do want to do is reclaim the human qualities culturally labeled 'male' and integrate them with the human qualities that have been seen as female so that we can all be fuller human people. This should also have the effect of freeing men from the pressure of being masculine at all times—a role equally as limiting as ours has been. We want, in short, to create a cultural environment where all qualities can come out in all people."

There is a general sense in which men and women need the strength characteristic of each other, both within themselves and in relationship to those of the opposite sex. Sensitivity, empathic understanding, intuitiveness, nurturance, and tenderness complement masculine traits both from within and from without. Such attributes, as already discussed, contribute to a personal wholeness, but they also contribute to interpersonal fulfillment and to completeness in pairing. Both the man and the woman want not only to feel love and understanding from one another, but also want to be proud of one another. The woman wants to feel and have acknowledged by her mate the value of the tasks she is able to accomplish. Such mutuality seems much more complete than the traditional view that the woman wants to hear "I love you" from her mate, while the man wants to hear "I'm proud of you" from his. Additionally, the woman who understands some of the strivings for competence, achievement, and assertion of her spouse through relating these issues within herself makes a better mate than the all-girl girl, just as the feeling man is a better partner than the man's man. In the Buddhist tradition, religious paintings and stories almost always include a goddess as part of the godhead, for without a goddess the god is incomplete, and lacks creativity and the ability to act.

When women find no in-the-world outlet for their legitimate strivings for expression of competence, achievement, and assertion, these qualities can emerge in a destructive sort of intramarital competition. If a woman depends entirely on a man to validate her sense of competence and ability, she may resent him, even unconsciously, for this power which, ironically, she herself has bestowed on him.

Just as the male can chase fantasies in the illusive pursuit of masculine identity, so can women have pseudo-identities based on defenses and secondary integrations that limit them as women and as people.

## *The Amazon*

"Men are fucked up! All they want from women is one thing. Who needs them anyway?" Some women, in seeking strength and in rejecting dependency on the male, seek or try to prove him superfluous, except perhaps reluctantly for breeding. A woman like this is the mirror image of the man who sees a woman only as a sex object and who may have contributed to creating her attitude in the first place. She likely saw her mother in a masochistic position, exploited and dominated by her father. She rejected identifying with her mother because of her weakness and resented her father for his inhumanity. Inevitable exposure during adolescence with guys on the make reinforced this perception of men. Annie's gun-brandishing song, "I can do anything you can do better, I can do anything better than you" epitomizes the Amazon's viewpoint. Peacetime contact with the Woman's Army Corps, for example, has indicated (GFS) that there appeared to be two conflicting motivations within the dominant WAC subculture, the first being to be as independent as possible from men, the second being to be "one of the boys." The WAC's ran their own mess halls, drove trucks, had their own military police, sought female military doctors, and even wanted a female chaplain (of whom there were none in the Army). Particular prestige was associated with competence in pistol shooting, team sports, and even, in one instance, in flame-throwing. On the other hand, a frequent comment, reflecting an intrinsic disparagement of women and an identification with a pejorative male chauvinistic view of femininity was, "You'd be nuts, too, Doc, if you had to live with a bunch of bitches."

A current manifestation of a similar process occurs among those women's rights activists who seek the exclusivity of an all-female society like that of a priesthood or an army, reflecting not a unique feminine identity, but an underlying envy of and identification with chauvinistic aspects of many men. They are the counterpart of traditional all-male groupings commented upon in Lionel Tiger's *Men in Groups*.

The Amazon is not necessarily overtly homosexual, nor does she promote "unisex" in the sense that it represents an equality and lack of differentiation between the sexes, but rather she is a female monosexist. A well-known woman active in the women's rights movement recently admitted a scathing self-criticalness and sense of weakness for having become hung up on a charming, handsome guy. She seemed to herself less of a person, as if something had been taken from her (her pseudo-autonomy?), rather than her life having been enriched by heterosexual mutuality.

### The Southern Belle

Just as the Amazon is the mirror image of the male chauvinist pig, the Southern Belle is the analog of the tough guy. Her hyperfemininity compares with his hypermasculinity. Not only does she have difficulty opening a car door, she swoons in the face of reptiles, rodents, and spiders. She confuses being a woman with being a child. She wants a daddy to take care of her, just as the house slaves waited on the mistress of the ol' manse. Physical effort is seen as unladylike, as is perspiring. Her husband may resort to the whorehouse for real sex. Gentility is confused with gentleness. She is likely to have had parents who undermined any assertive, competitive, or athletic strivings as unfeminine; she was likely to have been kept in crinoline and not permitted denims. She meets her aggressive and hostile needs through passive maneuvers. Her sick headaches have her husband by the balls. She seeks power through weakness. She both disguises and expresses her ("masculine") strivings for dominance by her hyperfemininity. She is not a woman because she is not a person. She is not a good mother because she still is a child herself.

### The Black Widow

The downfall of many a male has been the so-called "hysterical acting-out character." She is charming, attractive, flattering, and obstensibly sexy. Her basic motivations are to get and, at all costs, to be in control. Her male counterpart is likely to be a con man or wheeler-dealer. She uses her sexuality in the service of her narcissistic aims. She is basically cold and sexually dissatisfied. She is also competitive with the man and is a "ball breaker." After she marries her prey, she accuses him of unmanliness and undermines all his assertive attempts. She seeks weak men, while having fantasies of being overpowered by a dominant man, of whom she is really afraid. She may provoke her passive husband until he finally strikes her, until he proves her view of men as brutal, the classical wife-beater's wife. She is more concerned with the getting than the having and may need conquests to prove to herself her femininity, about which she is insecure, and to seek her insatiable desire to get. As a child, her basic needs for emotional nurturance ("orality") were either relatively unmet or she was overindulged—"spoiled" (itself a violation of basic maturation needs)—so that she never learned to tolerate frustrations of narcissistic demands. She did not develop adequate basic trust in others in terms of their reliability, on the one hand, or their ability to be in benevolent control on the other. The seductress uses her sexuality not to relate to men, but to win out over them.

Just as her hypothetical brother did not find father a suitable identification figure, she was not likely to have admired her father as a model of a desirable sex object. Her own basic needs were met through manipulation of her parents rather than through their understanding and spontaneous actions. Her mother may have been a similar classical "bitch."

This pattern may be attractive to many girls because of its glamor and "success." However, the seductress winds up as lonely as the black widow spider. The need to be in control is not a reflection of strength, but rather of insecurity. She has few women friends because she is competitive with women and basically distrusts them. Moreover, women are more likely to see through her than are men.

### The Prom Queen

The classical prom queen or pompom girl is the counterpart of the "big man on campus." She is a caricature of traditional middle-class cultural ideals, and appears to be becoming a rarer species except in her residual middle-aged form. (The hip chick is likely to have rejected the plasticity of her mother, class of '51.) The prom queen is a sex symbol without being genuinely sexual. Her responses are stereotyped and conventional. She knows how to be popular, but not how to be intimate. She is often admired and envied by other girls who are less attractive, less "in." She is a model toward which many girls strive. Yet, in tending to rely on her superficial but engaging social skills, her invariably good looks, she does not have to build a sense of self based on mastered challenges and surmounted hardships. Lacking the necessity, deeper inner strength is not typically cultivated. In later years, with fading beauty, she may have fewer and fewer friends and be quite lonely. Many of her less attractive sisters, having overcome the handicap of less physical beauty, having cultivated the ability to share more deeply and engage in intimate, abiding relationships, having perhaps developed their competence in a career or avocation, grow to be ever more attractive and interesting persons. The prom queen is similar to the all-American boy, Grinker's aforementioned "homoclite." She travels a well-worn path, is popular in school; she marries the boy next door who played baseball with dad, went to State

University, and came back to join his father's firm. Male or female homoclites are likely to fare poorly under stress when the chips are down. Not having had to overcome great obstacles, not having much practice at dealing with hardship and novelty, they often lack strength. Not having had to look to inner resources for success and interpersonal popularity, they also lack the inner awareness characteristic of the strong person. As the traditional middle class changes into new types of conventionality, the plastic dolly can be expected to assume new forms.

### The Happy Hooker

Just as the conquering Don Juan is a masculine fantasy, often sought for, rarely attained (and often unfulfilling when attained), so too is the happy hooker an archetypal fantasy in some young women. The appeal of lots of money, pleasure, conquest, associating with the most interesting of men, nice clothes, a beautiful apartment, calling your own shots, all amounts to an almost irresistible package. "Why should I be some man's secretary for $150 a week when I can make that much off the same man in a night, and with me being in charge, to boot." (The happy hooker fantasies leave out the pimp, to whom most real prostitutes relate in a dependent, highly exploited, and masochistic way.)

Just as much of the Don Juan's time is spent in exploitation of women, so too is the life of the happy hooker spent exploiting men. Although this life style may be both exciting and even fun, it is rarely fulfilling. For some, it may be a viable life'style; for most it is a fantasy that can never be attained. Just as the vast majority of women can never be a *Playboy* centerfold (posed, powdered, and touched up before being presented to the world), the life of the happy hooker is far beyond the reach of most women, except in fantasy. Both men and women can waste much time in pursuit of an unattainable fantasy, never to reach it, or on "reaching" it only finding it not what was dreamed. As already pointed out, fantasy is meaningful as preparation for reality; limiting when a substitute for it.

Again, as with other fantasies previously mentioned, trying to be something outside yourself, trying to make yourself in someone else's image, denies your own self; the path to meaning is in the wrong place, outside rather than inside. Especially when the fantasy being pursued does not contain elements of commitment, deep sharing and involvement, continuity of relatedness and learning the skills for developing genuine intimacy, the fantasy may become a dead-end street. When beauty fades, when you can no longer trade on your body and your youth, life may easily become empty unless these other skills have been developed. The exploiter then frequently becomes the exploited. The happy hooker may take the form of the gay divorcee, piling divorce settlement upon divorce settlement until the gigolo marries her, aging and sagging, and squanders the wealth earned through her years of courtesanship.

### *The Mother's Influence*

The role of the mother is perhaps even more critical for the girl than for the boy. Although Freud felt that the girl had the more difficult psychosexual task in switching from a homosexual (mother) to a heterosexual object relationship, we feel that, rather, the issue of identification is the more critical. The boy must switch from allegiance to the primary object, the nurturant mother, to the father as an identification figure, while the girl's primary relationship and identification figure can healthily remain the same. On the other hand, the mother, no matter how well she has functioned in that role, is frequently an inadequate model for the girl interested in instrumental skills, wishing to achieve outside the home or desiring a career that is meaningful for her rather than engaged in primarily to enhance family income. While the developing girl may be handicapped in assertive and achievement strivings and in outer mastery, she typically has an advantage over the boy in terms of inner and interpersonal masteries in that it is culturally permitted for her to show physical affection, to be emotionally responsive, to cry. Her feminine intuitiveness is seen as compatible with receptivity, and there are fewer social pressures for its repression.

Both for cultural reasons and because of their tendency to be more accepting of their own feelings, women are more apt to be in touch with and have less conflict about any fundamental bisexuality. For example, it has been reported that the female partners of most swinging couples engage in some homosexual activity, while manifest homosexual contact between the males is very rare. Another factor that may play a role in the prohibition of male but not female homosexuality has been the importance of desexualization of male-male bonding in cultural evolution. (Priesthoods of the past, armies, and current fraternal societies all meet their needs for affectional grouping of males, but simultaneously deny overt homosexuality.) Women have less tendency for such all-female groupings, a fact that is perhaps related to their lessened opportunity for peer groups such as those commonly found in pre-adolescent boys: "cops and robbers" or "cowboys and Indians," the neighborhood gang, Little League, and so forth. As such, pressures for desexualization of female-female relationships may be less and needs for emotional contact with the same sex more unmet.

### Women at Work

There is no doubt that for women as a group to develop their strength, they must have greater opportunities to be self-actualizing in trades and professions. Women as people, in addition to needing the chance to develop inner strength, need the opportunity for greater outer mastery. The world of work has placed severe limits on woman's opportunities for developing this. It is not our aim to add unnecessarily to the mounting number of dissertations written to justify the woman's right to work equally with men. In our minds, that this is needed for the increased development of strength is beyond serious debate. We feel it would be helpful, however, to point out some of the lesser known but still important pitfalls for women entering the occupational arena.

Beyond the rationalized arguments and fierce resistance of many a man against a woman's working alongside (not to mention above) him, are often strong, usually unconscious, resistances to a woman's working. In Pat Howe's words, "An example out of my own experience occurred when I was absent from my office for a substantial period of time because of illness. Working for me were many quite experienced, highly paid, and intelligent men. I had felt no trepidation in leaving the office in their capable hands. Yet I found in being absent that questions from the staff followed me in my absence. My staff had become very dependent upon me and my presence in the office, more so than they would have for a male boss. I had overlooked the fundamental ambivalence that men have in working for a woman. Men, even as adults, still want the protection and security they once had in their all-providing mother. Much of this need for protection and being taken care of and being dependent is missed in adulthood. Men both want and fear dependency. Working for a woman seemed to stimulate this fundamental ambivalence, especially because I believe I have been able to retain qualities of nurturance, affection, and caring so often associated with a maternal figure." Studies have shown that the most successful women in business are ones who have integrated their outer mastery with their supportive, nurturing selves. Thus, many men stalwartly resist women in work, not so much for the rational reasons so often heard, but often because it threatens to confront them with unresolved conflicts within themselves.

To continue with Pat Howe's observations, "A second incident in my career in the financial world revealed to me another roadblock to woman's working. I had been fortunate to have been quite successful in financial ventures, gaining the admiration of many men but arousing the suspicions and envy of many more. After having landed a particularly lucrative contract from a major governmental body, I was accused of having seduced a key man in the organization granting the contract. My picture appeared on the front page of a local paper with the incriminating accusations. So plausible was the charge that a regulating agency investigated my firm in the matter. I had encountered in a clear way what I had vaguely been aware of, namely: a common and deeply ingrained prejudice that the primary way a woman gets ahead is through her sexuality. Previously, it had been only an abstract understanding that men commonly treat women as sex objects."

Because so many men relate to women so simplistically, because so many men blindly assume that women's functions are primarily sexual and maternal, they often do not even comprehend that a woman may be an intelligent, efficient, well-organized individual. Because so many have the image of females primarily as potential sexual objects, often parents rear their daughters exclusively for this role, fearing their failure to capture and keep a mate. Girls then come to see themselves in the same limited way. A significant block to self-actualization through means other than the traditional feminine role ensues. Only recently have there evolved significant visible advocates of woman's right to actualize through development of competence in career and work choices. These people are providing the beginnings of an altered self-image for women. No longer is it necessary by default to accept the cultural norm that rewards only the sexual, maternal female (within marriage only, of course!). Additionally, this pattern has been difficult to break because of its previous evolutionary significance for the survival of the species. The maternal bond and the sexual bond with the male ensured the preservation of the species. Yet former evolutionary adaptations do not determine what makes for currently adaptive patterns. Change has been the hallmark of evolution, and the time seems ripe for further change in the male-female-sexual-work relationships.

Increasing the quality of life is becoming more of a goal than previously. In this sense, much of mankind is ready to raise its collective developmental level. The development of strength in women is an important part of this process. Quality has become more important as survival has become less of a daily issue. The evolution of woman to higher levels of developmirth (as is also true of men) will raise the collective consciousness to higher levels, a significant step forward, to be encouraged rather than fought.

The further concern that a successful working woman is intrinsically a less than adequate mother is not borne out by research studies. Stanley Coopersmith found that mothers who enjoy working are likely "to have children that are high rather than low in their self-esteem and are less likely to manifest anxiety and psychosomatic symptoms. The significance of the mother's absence from home apparently depends upon how she, her child, and the other members of the family view such absence. . . ."

Pat Howe: "I have more than once been disappointed at the results of the conflict between the maternal-familial needs and the desire to develop competence in the business world. I have long had the desire to groom competent women to function at the executive level in the financial world. I even subsidized a promising candidate at a graduate school of business. While working for me, she had said she was dedicated to having a career, determined never to allow home or family to interfere with her commitment to actualizing within the world of work. Yet within three years after obtaining her degree and returning to work with me in the firm, she finally could not maintain the two worlds and chose to return exclusively to the familial-maternal role. In its narrow sense, she could not see how such needs can be met in vocational ways or how both roles could be integrated. Such experiences, of course, reinforce the resistance to accepting women in professional schools and advanced training programs. Although more and more women are working, although expectations are changing, it is still difficult to find a great number of women able to combine domestic and, particularly, maternal roles with demanding competitive occupation. New models of role- and task-sharing within the home may prove helpful."

### Men Write Books—Women Have Babies

Productivity and creativity among men may be substitutes for rearing children. For women, generativity and even immortality may be met more directly through childbirth and child-rearing. Men miss this kind of creative experience. For many men, their creative outlet comes through an avocation. A history professor mentioned how upset he was that his wife never took the time to read the book he had just written: "You know, she has had babies; all I have had is my book." The total creative potential involvement in having children often competes favorably for a woman's time and energies with work and a career. The rearing of children, of course, can be a creative enterprise for either a man or a woman, and rearing children does not have to be a 24-hour job. Many men often strongly resist taking an equal or even a sharing hand in rearing their children, in their early years especially. Not only is this because of deeply ingrained cultural expectations, but also because at some level it is like messing in someone else's painting, like following the lead of someone else in finishing their project. To illustrate this bias, a well-respected child psychiatrist, when asked about the father's role during the child's first year of life, replied, "Keeping the mother happy." Not that these attitudes are justifications—it is just that they form part of the resistance in the man for trading his own little creative bailiwick (work) for that of someone else. Men often want to have "their own thing," as do women, and often resent and envy women for wanting the best of both worlds. If a good case can be made for "penis envy" among women, an equally plausible case can be made for "uterus envy" among men. Recognizing many of the unconscious resistances that men have against women's working makes it easier to cope with them to foster change and to enrich the lives of both women and men.

### Vicarious Living

A trap lurks behind fulfillment in motherhood—namely, that of the mother's living vicariously through her children because of the lack of direct satisfactions in her own life, other than that of the maternal role. Of course, this vicariousness can also exist in relationship to a husband's career. Such situations are optimal for neither person. In such a symbiosis, the one needs the other in order to be fulfilled and the other's accomplishments are not just for their own sake, but to please and gratify. Some women fulfill their own potentialities only when they are no longer needed to assist the development of their husband's and children's careers. Though late is better than never, it seems a shame that direct gratification of one's own talents need to be held so long in abeyance. The authoress of several best-selling, critically acclaimed novels began to write in her mid-fifties—only after her youngest son had married and obtained an academic appointment. She previously had contributed significantly to the professional development of her husband, younger brother, and older son.

## The Fruits of Overlapping Roles

Many side benefits, in fact, will accrue to both men and women as women in general become more integrated into the business and professional worlds. A common product of the current sharp division between the male provider and the female housewife is that the woman is not given an opportunity to develop interests and knowledge of those parts of the world that are important to her husband. He cannot share with his wife that which cannot be understood and appreciated. So often in such cases, the secretary becomes a surrogate wife to touch on the work-creative side of the man. (We have National Secretaries' Week. Mothers only get a day!) Just as a mother needs to share the importance of her day and relationships with the growing children with her husband, so, too, does the man need to talk about and have appreciated his efforts in his work. A secretary, co-worker, or female colleague, already sharing in this important part of his life, is often turned to for this needed intimacy and sharing. This is not to put all the blame on the wife's lack of interest for her husband's running around with his secretary, for it is in part he who put his wife in that position in the first place. The more the lives of women and men are integrated, the more the intimacy that can be shared meaningfully between them.

### Femininity

A feminine woman is conventionally defined as passive, receptive, intuitive, emotional, pacific, sensitive, fickle, understanding, and nurturing, but not as dominant, assertive, and worldly. Women must contend with the same problems with the concept of femininity as do men with the concept of masculinity. Just as masculinity can be a vague concept toward which men strive, never arriving, usually falling short, so it is with femininity. In striving to become something one is not, one's own experience is often denied, one's ability to affirm one's own person diminished.

Old distinctions, for example, are often limiting for a woman, such as the distinction claiming that women are passive and receptive while men are active and intrusive. Much of the support for this kind of distinction comes from the notion forcefully made popular by Freud that anatomy is destiny. Because the woman must receive a man sexually seemed to imply that she was therefore passive and receptive. Perhaps Freud had never been seduced by a sexually assertive woman. Perhaps Freud, a true Victorian, never had sex with an aroused and sexually responsive and eager woman at a time when he was tired and just wanted to enjoy himself passively while she actively pleased herself as well as him! Just as a woman may be limited in her sexual responsiveness by her conception of her role as passive, so too may a man be limited in his breadth of sexual pleasure by not allowing himself a view of a man as being sometimes passive and receptive. Thus, to distinguish or mark a woman as passive and a man as active is to draw analogies from anatomy and physiology that not only are inaccurate but also may be limiting to full expression (and full development) of both men and women.

Though some of us accept the utility of psychological-biological analogies, we often misread them. Certainly, such seems the case with feminine passivity. Obviously, the female is not necessarily passive during intercourse, though receptive. The primary analogy is that of union and cooperation. Both partners give of themselves and express their vulnerability. In psychosexual differences, we complement each other, and in a total expression of our overall human qualities are we most fulfilled.

### Expanded Visions of Womanhood

One virtue of the women's liberation movement is that it expands the horizons of a woman's possible conception of herself. The way one views oneself can be either limiting or expanding. Women's liberation has done much to begin to break down old limiting stereotypes through public forums, new books, news coverage, consciousness-raising sessions, lobbying for women's rights legislation, and so on. The changes being wrought are both exciting and broadening—and frightening, for any change is met with some ambivalence. As Joy and David Rice point out, "the appeal of woman's liberation to a woman's sense of dignity and the possibility of enhanced self-esteem . . . are very powerful attractants; indeed, the potential gain is often seen by many women as outweighing major initial risks, e.g., feelings of greater frustration with their lives, increased anger toward men, and the need for significant restructuring of their basic relationships with men." As has been mentioned, some women's liberationists, unfortunately, merely substitute an archaic view of the achieving aggressive male for the archaic view of the passive female. There is danger for the woman, as there is in other ways for the man, in defining self-esteem by what one does. We feel it is important for women to enter the traditional masculine working world bringing with them their own values. When they begin to define their self-worth in terms of paychecks and power structures, they have lost the enriching perspective that women can contribute.

Current changes and challenges and broadened horizons are creating new problems for the identity formation of women. No longer is there a clear and simple feminine ideal with which to contend. No longer is a woman limited to being a housewife, mother, secretary, nurse, or schoolteacher. The strong woman will explore more and more avenues, seeking to express herself, finding more paths open for such expression in a world formerly populated only by men. She has more ambiguity and uncertainty with which to contend. Yet she will do so not denying her fundamental biological and psychological womanhood, but finding new ways of affirming and integrating her femaleness into new areas of competence and worldly skill. Less inclined to be limited by either old or new conceptions of actual femininity, she will attempt to affirm and relate to her own unique experience, actualizing herself rather than others' image of or wishes for her. She will have much the same attitude about her experience and womanhood as stated by Ingrid Bengis: "The only thing I'm militant about is the necessity for struggling to be as fully human as we can." The affirmation of and growth from one's own unique experience, whether one is man or woman, is one of the central traits of the strong person. A woman must try to create herself using her own awareness of inner experience rather than trying to become someone else's definition of what a woman is "supposed" to be. As Ms. Bengis has resolved for herself, "I cannot be the completely feminine woman of the '50s, the sexually free woman of the '60s and the militant, anti-sexist woman of the '70s. I cannot ignore the fact that my own life has unfolded slowly, that it has been a part of all those trends and none of them." She has instead come to see herself as uniquely Ingrid, a contemporary person who terms herself a "Puritan romantic." She is what she is choosing to be, based on her own self-understanding. Such is the course of a strong woman.

# PART THREE:

## Interpersonal Mastery

# 4

# STRENGTH AND INTIMACY

Closeness, intimacy, love, sharing—so wished for, so talked about—are rarely achieved. Intimacy appears deceptively easy to come by. Yet the road to genuine intimacy is fraught with risks, dangers, and obstacles often perceived as so great that many fear achieving the very quality of life they value and long for most. One of the central manifestations of strength is in the ability to create and sustain intimacy with others. As Joseph Simon and Jeanne Reidy point out in *The Risk of Loving*, each of us longs "to share the joy and the sorrow, the depression and the bliss, the experiences which give life real meaning. We want to reveal that inner self we keep too meticulously hidden." We all experience moments when we want to be held and taken care of, when we want someone else to minister to our needs. We want to value and be significant to some others and to have such others be significant to us. These feelings are real and human. They are feelings that need to be acknowledged and understood in ourselves. To be intimate requires that such legitimate strivings be shared with another. Desmond Morris in *Intimate Behavior* says that, contrary to popular apprehensions, "the soothing and calming effects of gentle intimacies leave the individual freer and better equipped emotionally to deal with the more remote, impersonal moments of life. They do not soften him, as has so often been claimed, they strengthen him, as they do with the loved child who explores more readily."

Within every person is a rich and vast potential: wide ranges of emotional life (anger, joy, resentment, love, hate, tenderness, rage, affection, sorrow), intricate and fascinating fantasies (of success, of sexual intrigue, of strange and wonderful experiences), complex and obscure dreams (often suggestive, but not quite understandable, both expressing and disguising wishes or fears, and occasionally frightening in their clarity), and a myriad of thoughts and creative urges. The individual is most apt to know and to experience himself fully when he has shared fully with another. When someone else knows you as well as you seem to know yourself, you begin to know yourself even better.

### Intimacy as Sharing

Total intimacy involves sharing yourself without reservation, not as a compulsive or absolution-seeking confession but out of a desire to be open, whole, and honest. Sharing completely does not mean sharing selectively. Many would prefer to think of being intimate as sharing only the acceptable and positive: joy, love, tenderness, and affection, for example. But intimacy is the sharing of all your experience. It is giving the gift of yourself—all of yourself. Intimacy requires exposure of oneself, the embarrassing as well as the conventionally valued.

The ability to share yourself does not imply the loss of self or of individual boundaries. Whatever the degree of communication, of empathy, and understanding of how another feels, one is not another. I may understand and share your feelings, but we are not tuning forks of an identical frequency, vibrating together. I am myself. I use my humanness to reverberate with yours, but at some level must face an existential loneliness, for some aspects of me are unique and separate, perhaps not even completely understood.

An example comes to mind involving what could be called pseudo-intimacy. As a young teacher, I (GFS) was asked to supervise a buxom middle-aged psychiatric social worker, about whose professional training and experience I knew nothing. Upon our meeting, I asked her for some information about her background. She quickly replied, "I loathed my mother. I had an incestuous fixation on my father. For many years I was extremely promiscuous. Now I have a semi-satisfactory marriage." I interjected, "No, no, no. Where did you go to school?" Needless to say, we never became intimate.

Today, while beginning to work on this chapter, an intern with whom I had some experience as a teacher was being interviewed for the psychiatric residency of which I'm in charge. He seemed different from my prior impression of him as a bigoted, aggressive, even somewhat hostile young man. He was gentle, his eyes expressive. He told of his awe, fear, and respect of me, his past searches for a hero, his current wish to find realistic models as well as of the personal and sexual fulfillment he is finding in his second marriage in which he is avoiding the mistakes of the first. I countered with my own futile quests for heroes, warning him against trying to make one of me. It was an intense encounter. I allowed myself to react and decide intuitively—he has the residency. He said "I have a feeling you're going to be more than my teacher. We're going to be friends!" I believe him.

## *"Love Thyself as Thy Neighbor"*

Self-intimacy and shared intimacy go hand in hand. In order to share one's own complex experience, there must be a sensitive listening ear to those sometimes quiet voices that tell of our own inner experience. To varying degrees, many of us are fearful of, deny, turn away from, or hide many of our thoughts and feelings from conscious awareness. To the extent that this is true, we have not achieved communion with ourselves. The depth and richness of our intimate experiences with others are directly limited by the fullness of, our knowledge of, and our caring for our own personal experience. We are dishonest with others when we are dishonest with ourselves. Some feel as guilty for what they feel as for what they do, and then devote much psychological energy to the repression of any unacceptable thought or emotion. Such people are constricted and have fewer resources in their present lives, so much effort being expended in "rear-guard" actions. We are responsible for our behavior. We need not control our thoughts. A sexual or aggressive fantasy *per se* never hurt anyone else. The strong person differentiates between thought and action—not so the obsessive, who must ward off unacceptable thoughts like deeds, or the psychopath, who acts on whatever impulse he has or can get away with. A strong person can judge whether acting on motives is appropriate, can evaluate their possible consequences in terms of both conscience and reality, and behaves accordingly.

## *Intimacy as Touching*

Most people in our culture find great difficulty in sharing their bodies. Although basic needs for nongenital touch and physical contact are being increasingly documented, the descriptions of America, with its Northern European Anglo-Saxon cultural past, as an anti-touch culture are also escalating. Desmond Morris defines intimacy as body contact. In asserting the need for touching, he says, "Perhaps touch is so basic—it has been called the mother of senses—that we tend to take it for granted. Unhappily, and almost without our noticing it, we have gradually become less and less touchful, more and more distant, and physical untouchability has been accompanied by emotional remoteness. It is as if the modern urbanite has put on a suit of emotional armor and, with a velvet hand inside an iron glove, is beginning to feel trapped and alienated from the feelings of even his nearest companions."

William E. Hartman notes that so pervasive is our aversion to touching in affectionate ways that even nudist colonies have typically adopted no-touch rules in the past. Although nudists share their bodies visually one with another, he believes "much more personal growth would take place among individuals where there is some kind of affectionate touch contact, especially with closely related individuals and generally between all persons." The need for body contact between persons is so important that Ashley Montagu has written an entire book *(Touching)* concerning our deep-seated needs for touch. He summarizes much of the evidence indicating the great need of infants for body contact and stimulation, saying that what the child needs for proper growth and a healthy emotional life is to be touched, handled, caressed, and cuddled. Extreme deprivation of these needs leads to the well-known *marasmus effect,* in which infants may actually die for lack of bodily stimulation even in the face of adequate nutrition and shelter.

People tend to extrapolate the degree of distance they experienced in a primary parental relationship (generally mother-child) into subsequent relationships. Depending upon the degree of closeness with which one is familiar and comfortable, one may pursue those who flee and flee those who pursue, always thus maintaining considerable interpersonal distance. Some cultures, particularly those of Northern Europe, foster distance and no-touch; others, particularly of the Pacific Islands, foster closeness and contact. There are even considerably different preferred distances for standing during conversation among cultures.

There tends to be a subtle belief, even among those who know that children need to be held and touched, caressed and patted, that these needs are outgrown and are no longer important for an adult. Yet Morris points out that in the adult world, filled with stress, anxieties, and frustrations, we often want to reach out, we do hunger for the direct and meaningful expression of affection and caring that is best communicated through touch. But so often do others fail to respond to our need that "we are in danger of becoming starved of the primary reassurance of bodily contact. . . . We are liable to become touch hungry and body-lonely." A business executive, asked how he met his needs for being touched and held, responded: "What do you think I am! I'm no kid anymore." The subject was dropped as we went on to talk about his latest affair.

### "Second-Hand" Touching

With the absence of touch in everyday lives, it is not uncommon for people to find second-hand (so to speak) ways of meeting their needs for touch. Many avenues are formalized and ritualized: greetings, handshakes, pats on the back, the football hug, the playful tickling between friends. Morris speaks of "the professional touchers": the doctors, masseurs, shoeshiners, rubdowners, hairdressers, barbers, and tailors. Would it sound perverse to say that people are often more intimate with animals than with people? Perhaps, however, the needs for touching, cuddling, holding, and expressing affection are most easily expressed via the pet cat or dog, which is usually described as one of the family. Animals like to be held and touched and stroked; so do people. Research among nonhuman primates reveals that grooming behavior serves to establish and reinforce affectionate ties within a social group; its adaptive function is far greater than the mere removal of parasites and debris. Monkeys, cats, and dogs show their needs more directly. A man so hardened that he does not relate to anyone still may be able to give affection to his dog. The need is still there, even if the avenue to express it in relationship to other human beings is blocked.

Not meeting their needs for physical intimacy among friends, many turn to lovers, affairs—mistresses or masters. Montagu reports that many women entice men into sexual relationships by saying, "I just wanted to be held." "I just wanted someone to be close to." Even the prostitute (particularly the male hustler) may be rationalizing by ostensibly commercial motivations a need for closeness in the face of feared real intimacy. (How ironic that one may find sex acceptable for money, but not for closeness!) This pattern is not surprising, because our culture has made the unfortunate linkage of touching and body intimacy solely with sex. As early as the nineteenth century, the phrase "to be intimate" came to mean the same as to have sexual intercourse. Today, it is extremely difficult to have bodily contact between adults without sexual motivation being suspected or felt. So the circular problem develops wherein there is no touching without sexual motivation implied—most sexual contact is forbidden, so why touch in the first place? Consequently, many of us spend our daily lives with important needs going chronically unmet. (Of course, bodily contact can also have aggressive connotations; people touch when they fight except when fighting is depersonalized by modern technology— from handguns to atomic bombs.)

### Fear of Touching

As a psychiatric consultant to the Peace Corps, I (GFS) was involved in training programs for volunteers preparing to go to the Philippines. I routinely asked returned volunteers to discuss with trainees difficulties they had encountered in adjusting to the Philippine culture. Almost invariably, they cited physical contact among friends as anxiety-provoking. In the Philippines, male friends hold hands; female friends often kiss. Filipino males were outraged when sexual motives or effeminacy were implied by insensitive Peace Corps volunteers, and both men and women were offended by the aloof, "unfriendly" behavior of the Americans. Some volunteers came to accept and enjoy the physical demonstrativeness shown by Filipinos and became frustrated upon return to the more distancing American culture.

Misinterpretation or definition of touch as intrinsically sexual, fears of intimacy in general, and abhorrence of the sensual as bad or dirty all contribute to the avoidance of touching. Our culture defines a rather large "body buffer zone." Coming within it may seem as intrusive, as an invasion of territory, and may be perceived as either a sexual or an aggressive move. Every psychiatrist knows that a paranoid patient may attack if he gets too close; yet he should also know how a frightened, sad, or anxious patient may be calmed and comforted by a hand held, an arm around a shoulder, or even a head on one's shoulder.

Stating a problem, of course, does not necessarily imply its solution. More will be said about physical contact, however, in later chapters on the sexual dimension of physical intimacy, and some concrete suggestions of a positive nature made in the chapter on developing personal strength.

### Intimacy as Intercourse Not Masturbation

For genuine intimacy, far more than a physical dimension of experience is required. All you know of life and of the world about is based upon your own direct or indirect experience. There is an ultimate subjectivity that must be acknowledged. We relate to our experience of the world, of another person, rather than to the world or to another person directly. The less you are able to experience of yourself, the less you know of the world. Conversely, the less you share of yourself with another, the less you know of yourself.

One experiences himself differently in relationship to different people. With some, an individual may find a depth of seriousness in himself; with others, he may find his humor, a sense of joy or of peace. Different people touch on or bring an awareness of varying parts of your own experience. Those people who come to touch upon valued dimensions of your own experience thus become significant others; without them you would be deprived of some knowledge of yourself and the range of your own experiential potential. Intimacy enriches the experience of both persons in relationship to each other; the street must be two-way. Intimacy is, then, a means to personal growth and requires the direct participation of another. Growth involves intercourse and does not come from psychological masturbation. Although meditation may promote relaxation or extension of perceptivity, and introspection and reflection serve to integrate experience, a man or woman does not develop in isolation. As Martin Buber *(I and Thou)* and Joshua Heschel ("Existence is coexistence") have pointed out from a philosophic frame of reference and Joseph Solomon ("I am thought about, therefore I am") from a psychoanalytic, man's very sense of being or existence depends on interaction with significant others.

### Intimacy: A New Taboo

That the old Victorian taboo about explicit, frank, and open discussion of sexuality is gone need not be belabored. When "Nude Sex Therapies," with a picture of a naked young couple (albeit above the waist) is the cover story in a national news magazine, the point is self-evident. As a new taboo there has been a growing awareness of the subject of death as hidden and forbidden. Death generally takes place in sterile isolation and is disguised by the mortuary beautician, but this is another topic. Young people are free to discuss sex and, usually, to engage in sexual behavior. However, when they are frank, they often admit major problems in being intimate. As one student recently put it, "The only girl I really talk to is my room-mate's girl friend. I'm too busy making out with the chicks I date." He could open up to a "safe" girl, one with whom he could not be fully intimate. Sexuality was not the result of intimacy, or even a means toward it, but rather a defense against it.

A strong person is recognized in part by his ability to enter into and to sustain intimate relationships. He is able to risk exposing himself, the good and the bad, without fear of losing himself, without fear of being rendered helpless by rejection, and without fear of becoming dependent. He values all of his experience and sees the sharing of that experience with others as offering the gift of himself to another. It may seem silly to think that strength would be required for intimate behavior. Qualities like courage, risk-taking, and strength are usually reserved for men and women in the face of adversity or physical danger. Yet physical and emotional courage may be totally unrelated. The bruising line-backer, playing an entire game with a broken rib, may not be able to tell his girl friend that he truly needed her.

Why should intimacy, so sought after, be so feared? So afraid are we of genuine intimate contact that intimacy is the exception rather than the rule in our relationships. Intimacy is a normal but nonnormative aspect of our human experience. One surveyor of a college campus revealed that only 10 percent of "normal" students, those who had never received treatment for emotional problems, were capable of truly intimate ties with a friend or lover, while 20 percent of the "normal" students had diagnosable psychiatric disorders. (Thus, it may be hard for a strong person to find another as capable of intimacy as he or she.)

### Fear of Dependency

Courage is needed to confront the fears and problems associated with intimacy. Dependency is a problem for many. The clinging, dependent person is never truly intimate with the one upon whom he or she leans. Intimacy is a relationship between equals. Parent-child closeness is of another sort. The adult who is dependent on only one other is intrinsically ambivalent. The person without whom one cannot live is inevitably resented. While being grateful, the debtor usually resents his creditor and his own relatively inferior position. The mature and intimate relationship must be nonambivalent (which is not to say, of course, that no negative feelings ever arise in its context). The dependent person fears expression of any negative feelings because he can not tolerate rejection. Honesty thus becomes difficult. You dare not bite the hand that feeds you. Neither the superior nor the inferior (neither the master nor the slave) is a truly self-reliant person who can choose to enter into an intimate relationship with a peer. Each needs the other to complete his sense of self.

A most common barrier to intimate behavior is the fear of dependency. In a world that values independence, autonomy, self-sufficiency, the self-made man, "pulling yourself up by your own bootstraps," and being sure of oneself, to be dependent is to be weak. To be dependent is to regress, to backslide, to be vulnerable to rejection. Both those who are overtly dependent and those who fear dependency do not trust. The dependent person cannot let go because he does not see the world as predictable, reliable, and giving. Those who fear dependency cannot become involved because they cannot perceive another as accepting, consistent, and reliable.

In developmental terms, the groundwork is laid early for later problems of dependency. The infant's first move toward autonomy is usually with his thumb. The thumb in the mouth makes mother (or breast) less necessary. Winnicott refers to the security blanket and teddy bear as transitional objects aiding in moving a child from mother to other interpersonal relationships. Joseph Solomon, rather, sees these as substitute objects. He points out that dependency can be not only on people but upon fixed ideas or fixed repetitive patterns of behavior, which represent such substitute objects and thus serve as surrogates for mother. Such varied forms of dependency arise either from the frustration of basic needs or from failure at individuation and maturation. Those who cling obsessively to ideas or compulsively to specific behavior patterns may avoid involvement with people, who are seen as less reliable than their substitutes. Such patterns are thus analogous to addiction. Just as the junkie is concerned with his fix, not with relationships, the person with fixed ideas or behavior patterns is preoccupied with his concept of being special or bad or whatever, with gaining acceptance, or even provoking rejection, and, thus, with whatever has come to symbolize or substitute for the original mother-child union. Those who depend on substitute patterns may appear to be independent in relationship to other people. Those who fear dependency actually are most dependent.

Obviously, dependency is a normal phase of childhood development. The infant must be fed, held, and kept warm. Later, the child learns he can depend on his parents or their surrogates and does not need constant care and gratification. Ultimately, he learns that he can rely on himself to meet his own needs in the world and with others.

Those afraid of relating often must go through similar phases of dependency, interdependency, and ultimate self-reliance and trust in order to achieve maturity. Fears of the initial dependency interfere with the establishment of such needed relationships, including that with a psychotherapist—"transference resistance." Under stress, there is often a regression to a more dependent and infantile stage. We all know how much we want to be taken care of when we are sick and frightened. Even the strongest person is not completely free of dependency needs, especially in times of crisis. A sign of strength, indeed, is the ability to accept and express these needs at such times.

### Fear of Merging, Loss of Self and of Identity

Even more primitive than the fear of dependency is the fear of merging, or loss of self. When one is unsure of himself, when he does not know where he stands in life, when he is chronically vague and ambivalent about himself, his values, his feelings (when he has poor ego boundaries), then he may avoid intimacy for fear of being engulfed or overwhelmed. He may fear losing what little of certainty and stability there is in himself. Where boundaries are vague and weak, they may not survive contact or buffeting. He fears loss of self either through engulfment by the other person or by his own emotions as engendered by the other person.

The expressions are often heard: "I can't be myself around him (or her)," or "I am afraid of being overpowered by him." Both bespeak a fear of merging, loss of self, or loss of ego boundaries. In the words of Thomas Harris, the strong person is better able to say to himself, "I am O.K. The feelings I have are me, no matter how weird or unacceptable to others, and it is O.K. for me to have them. I am interested in myself, my feelings, my thoughts and my fantasies for they are real parts of my experience of life. I take responsibility for what I do and how I behave, but I do not feel guilty for nor do I try to control what I feel. Accepting my own feelings, others then cannot make me feel too bad for having them by playing on my own guilt about them. I am not confused about where my feelings end and another's begin."

Having this attitude, you can share of yourself more fully. Not being ashamed of your own feelings, being willing to take responsibility for your own feelings, and being able fully to experience them without disintegration, you can enter more completely into a relationship without fear of losing yourself. A strong person is not a chameleon taking on the coloring of his surroundings. He can shift roles without losing his identity. Though he behaves differently in different situations and in relationship to different people, he is always himself. He takes suggestions without being suggestible.

The person with a very rigid sense of identity may fear loss of self in intimate relationships. Being intimate includes revealing anxieties and troubles and admitting needs. The rigid appearance presented by the authoritarian father or the well-structured friendliness of the social butterfly are really facades covering numerous natural and human (although feared and labeled as being unacceptable) feelings. Because their identity is so firmly bound up with the facade presented to others, intimacy threatens their sense of self, for it would require losing the front. The fear of losing a sense of oneself, of being cast adrift without a helmsman, is frightening, so frightening that the facade is held onto for dear life. It is analogous to holding onto a piece of driftwood, which may have previously served to aid survival, when one is now able to stand up on the firm ground that is underfoot. The person then clings to archaic, maladjusting ways of gaining security rather than to real and satisfying means readily available—i.e., the sense of peace, wholeness, and security found in the truly intimate relationship. In the theological sense, one must be willing to die (in the sense of giving up a security device or a limiting conception of oneself) in order to be reborn (in the wholeness possible through intimacy both with God and with others). If one has not experienced the fullness of himself in intimate relationship with another, it requires some measure of faith to follow the lead of someone who beckons to a better place. When the fear transcends the faith and hope held out by intimacy, the person remains floating in the sea, going nowhere.

### Fear of Weakness

Weakness is taboo—or if not taboo, it is at least unmanly (and in terms of women's liberation, unwomanly, too). People who show weakness are labeled variously as creampuffs, fags, or sissies. Many believe a key sign of weakness is shown when one cannot control one's feelings, for "only weak people have no self-control." In many circles, the expression of feelings is directly associated with weakness. To be troubled or upset or uncool is to admit that you don't have control over yourself. This is considered weakness, lack of backbone, unmanly. A presidential candidate can lose his party's nomination for weeping publicly over published, falsely planted vilifications of his wife.

True courage or strength, however, consists not in "heroically" (more accurately, unhumanly) keeping feelings hidden. (Admittedly, however, the wise have the sense to control the expression of even appropriate emotions when their revelation would be misconstrued.) Rather, strength is demonstrated in accepting feelings and failures and lack of omnipotence as a real and acceptable part of yourself. The fear of confronting weakness in yourself is thus a block to intimacy. Strength is in allowing loss of control, but not in losing control, in admiting weakness, but in not being overwhelmed by inadequacy.

### Fear of Rejection, Hurt, Abandonment

Fears of rejection, hurt, and abandonment are other blocks to intimacy. For every exquisite pleasure there is the pain of not having that pleasure when it is gone. For every peak there may lie a valley beyond.

To love is to be lonely. Every love eventually is broken by illness, separation or death. The exquisite nature of love, the unique quality or dimension in its highest peak, is threatened by change and termination. All love leads to suffering. If we did not care for others in a deep and fundamental way, we would not experience grief when they are troubled or disturbed, when they face tragedy or misfortune, when they are ill or dying. Every person is ultimately confronted with the pain of separation of death, with tragic grief which can be healed in silence and isolation. (Moustakas)

Man avoids intimacy in order to avoid confronting the depths and power of his own loneliness and suffering. Rather, he chooses a very constricted life style, as in Paul Simon's ballad:

> I am a rock. I am an island.
> And a rock feels no pain and an island never cries.*

Fearing, rather than valuing deep bittersweet feelings, many people never allow themselves the richness of a loving, intimate relationship. A "biker" nicknamed "Harley," whose only love-object was his "chopper," revealed the motto of his motorcycle club as "Love slows you down." One who does not have cannot lose. Some avoid intimacy to avoid being hurt. Others avoid wanting intimacy for fear of not obtaining it.

### Fear of Wanting and Not Getting

The more fully aware of one's inner life, one's deeper needs and

---

* From "I Am a Rock," © 1965 Paul Simon. Used with permission of the publisher.

desires, the more one is aware of the extent of his need for human contact, warmth, and affection. To recognize the need may only compound the problem in the absence of knowing the skills and ways of relating that will bring about the wanted closeness. To recognize a want while not knowing how to get that want met is worse than denying that the want exists in the first place. In such a case, a drive itself becomes feared ("instinctual anxiety").

Much of what is described as neurotic behavior is a product of this very dilemma. The neurotic has a glimpse of what he wants from others in life, but does not know how to go about getting it. The ways in which he tries to express his needs are self-defeating and block his path rather than help him along it. His primary symptoms are inhibitions and anxiety, for he cannot figure out what he is doing wrong. His ways of warding off anxiety bring on new problems. His gloomy prophecies are self-fulfilling.

A middle-aged priest thinks of leaving the priesthood. He has come to discover in himself more fully than ever his tremendous needs for affection, caring, and physical contact that cannot be met in his role as a priest. Being a direct and honest person, he immediately tells others of his great feelings of liking and attraction toward them, and of his great need for affection. The others, feeling overwhelmed and fearing engulfment in the light of the power of his feelings, invariably back away from him. The priest is in touch with real needs in himself, but the way he relates his needs to others is self-defeating, for it does not elicit the affection that he so strongly desires in return.

To want, but not to know how to get or to have, is incredibly exasperating. Many choose to deny the want in order to avoid the frustration of not having. Sometimes, it must seem like a cruel joke perpetrated on mankind when intimacy, love, and affection should be so highly valued, yet their pursuit so frequently blocked.

To acknowledge the wants and needs for affection and intimacy, both physical and emotional, causes problems. Sharing more fully with others tends to elicit more feelings of closeness and attraction in them. Yet many of these feelings are bound to be frustrated in their full expression. You are drawn toward your neighbor's husband, your husband's best friend. You have come to be very close to your secretary, your wife's attractive little sister, your mother-in-law. For married persons, intimacy with those outside the marital relationship is typically forbidden, impractical, emotionally costly, threatening, destructive of the marriage, and so on. So, rather than go through the frustration of having wants and needs unfulfilled and a primary relationship threatened, many married people deny the want and often come to resent their marriages for limiting their ability to seek and fulfill genuine human needs for affection and caring. In the process, the dearth of intimacy is perpetuated.

### *Jealousy and Possessiveness*

Commitment to a partner, the primacy and special total nature of one relationship, does not imply that the needs and wishes for intimacy and meaningful inter*change* (not inter*course*) are necessarily met through that one relationship. Significant others enrich your experience, particularly when their friendship is mutually shared by both partners. No one owns another. Few emotions are as destructive as the selfishness of possessiveness. Those fearing rejection often thus provoke it and bring about their expectations, not their wishes. If one feels lovable, worthy, and valued and feels a commitment from his spouse, lover, or friend, he or she is not threatened by other relationships. Expecting all from one person places a burden on any relationship. Yet, intimate friendships need be few. There is neither time nor emotional energy for many. The strong person, capable of intimacy, must at times reject opportunities for close friendships, of which he or she might otherwise be capable, simply because of existing commitments.

Secondary relationships, with their opportunity to meet varied needs and to gain perspective on a primary relationship and provide outside help in the face of stress within it, tend to preserve the primary commitment. Such friendships, when shared with your lover, may enhance and enrich the primary relationship. They also sustain one in the face of the loss of a loved one.

### *Fear of Being Self-Conscious*

The depths and real rewards of intimacy come not with easy revelations of things one has done or said or thought or felt, not with the revelation of feelings or emotions that are familiar and acceptable to oneself, or with the parts of oneself with which one is comfortable and at home and can express with glibness and facility. Some people seem to be incredibly open because they can disclose things about themselves that seem quite revealing. Yet the revelations are so well in control, so familiar and accepted by the person, that the risk involved for him is not great at all. He has complete control over that part of himself.

It is easier to reveal something that one has mastery and control over than something that is troubling and half-formulated. It may be easier to reveal some thought or feeling from the past than one that is in the present, though the converse can also be true. It is easier to reveal to someone what you would like to feel toward him or would like to do with him than what you are feeling toward them in the present moment. It is easier to say in reference to yourself: "Well, you know, you feel bad sometimes," rather than "Well, I'm feeling pretty bad." The most difficult revelation for any of us and the most intimate at a given moment is what I am feeling about you right now. If the feeling is seen as having risk in the revelation or if the feeling is only half-formulated or obscure in one's own mind, the risk is enhanced. Whenever one relates to another beyond the clear understanding of his own feelings, the risk is increased. These kinds of revelations, this form of sharing, is avoided assiduously by most people. To reveal one's here and now, half-understood, half-formulated, somewhat unacceptable or embarrassing feelings, one must be self-conscious in the sense of being self-aware. The skilled psychotherapist knows that if a patient habitually talks about the present, he does not want to face traumatic memories, that if he continually talks about the past, there is a current conflict, that if he talks about both, he may be avoiding revealing feelings about the therapist. The patient who first discusses difficulty with his mother typically has an important problem with his father.

Many people oppose spontaneity and self-awareness. If asked, most people would probably say that they valued spontaneity. To be spontaneous means, for most, the expression of oneself naturally, without analytical thought or self-consciousness—to express oneself easily and fully without having to deliberately grope for the right words. If one is self-conscious, he considers himself no longer to be spontaneous. Self-consciousness, then, feels to most people as though they are being artificial. Being artificial carries many negative connotations, such as being unreal, plastic, not being worth very much. Thus, self-consciousness is often thought of as being unreal or as an undesirable state of affairs.

Yet, in truth, the times when one is most self-conscious are often times when one is being most real. The meaning of one's sharing is heightened because of the greater risk involved in revealing parts of oneself that are not under firm verbal and intellectual control. They are times of heightened self-awareness, of being more in touch with the range of oneself than one normally is. Rather than being confused by trying to be spontaneous at these moments, it is often more helpful to value oneself as being congruent. Being congruent means presenting on the outside what is going on inside you at the moment. One is being more real and more intimate at that moment by sharing rather than by hiding his self-consciousness.

It takes strength to be congruent. It means accepting oneself and self-revelation and thus risking possible rejection or misunderstanding. Even if a person becomes accepting of self-conscious involvement, others may not. They may run away or become angry or think one weird. Strength is being willing, however, to be as congruent as you can at any given moment, being willing to risk being self-conscious, to risk the possible rejection of others. This is most possible when you can accept and evaluate yourself, rather than letting the judgment of others ruin your self-esteem and self-concept. There is, of course, a needed balance between obliviousness to feedback and oversensitivity. The self-assured person is not complacent and uses intimacy to find directions for growth. If self-conscious relatedness is difficult between the sexes, it is often even more difficult for members of the same sex.

### Fear of Homosexuality

This fear, which prevents intimacy between members of the same sex, is found in both men and women, but is more pronounced in men. The greater the sharing between two people, the greater the emotional bond. The deeper the sharing, the stronger the feelings of affection and liking for the other. This is true whether the relationship is between a woman and a man or between two men or two women. Feeling affection and closeness is frightening between two men if it is expressed directly, for it immediately suggests the possibility of homosexual intent. For men, so many natural human feelings of interest, attraction, and affection are directly associated with being homosexual that any direct expressions of intimacy between men is typically avoided. Most men, for example, will not allow themselves to gaze in a shower room with aesthetic appreciation upon the body of another man. Only sideways glances are made toward the genitals of another. If you asked a man to try to understand the attractiveness of another man to a woman by looking at the man through a woman's eyes, you might get a fist in the mouth. A counselee confessed that she was afraid of being a lesbian and avoided looking at other women's breasts because she might find them attractive.

Both men and women can be attractive creatures in body and mind. The deeper the sharing between two persons, the deeper the affection and attraction. Emotional attraction between members of the same sex is often mistaken for homosexuality. Finding a person attractive is not the same as finding him or her sexually arousing. Homosexuality in males implies weakness and femininity and is thus more socially abhorred than it is among women, who, in chauvinistic terms, are "coming up in the world" if they have masculine behavior or strivings. Lionel Ovesey points out that fears of homosexuality in males may actually represent fears of weakness, dependency, and passivity rather than a concern about actual sexual impulses toward members of the same sex.

Friendship and intimacy with members of the same sex (*iso*sexual relationships) are enormously important and valuable. Perhaps it takes another man to understand the urgent nature of a young man's sexual drives or another woman to understand the peculiar irritability of premenstrual tension. Individuals of the same sex tend to "see through" the phoniness and pretensions of another member of the same sex, while the opposite sex is more easily seduced and duped. Perhaps useful advice might be, "Never date a girl without girlfriends or a boy without boyfriends." A person secure in his or her sexual identity feels comfortable with members of the same sex and is generally liked by them. After all, half the world consists of the same sex. (Many overt homosexuals make the reciprocal mistake; they fear not only sexual but emotional intercourse with the opposite sex.)

### *Fear of Risk*

To become intimate thus requires strength, because intimacy necessitates taking risks. Many people leave their lives up to chance. They wait for someone to come along who will appreciate them, who will show interest and caring by drawing them out, by passing through a gauntlet of barriers designed to keep others out except for the most persistent. Those who persist will pass a test and be allowed in. A tick lies patiently in a tree for months, waiting for a warm-blooded animal to pass beneath, at which time it drops, to lodge on the skin of the passing animal. If unsuccessful, it returns to its perch, again awaiting the chance encounter that will allow it to fulfill its destiny, that will keep it alive.

Those seeking and capable of intimacy best not wait for the knight in shining armor, best not leave life up to chance. The psychological risks of intimacy or of establishing intimate contacts are many and often far more frightening than physical danger: the risk of being misunderstood, the risk of being rejected, the risk of being not wanted or not desired. A champion weight-lifter can be scared of his wife.

Significant sharing involves giving a part of oneself into the hands of another, with the trust that he or she will cherish and "care carefully" for that precious gift.

Traditionally negative emotions can be shared too: anger, anxiety, depression, resentment, bitterness, and so on. The risks here likewise are great. The skill comes in having negative emotions without having to direct them, of feeling negative emotions without attacking with them. Some of the best friendships occur between those who once felt antagonism toward each other, but shared in that event. The risks are that the other will be defensive and withdraw, that the other person may dislike you for confronting him with troubling emotions, that the other person may only get angry and attack. In sharing negative feelings, it is important that the underlying good will come through. We do not refer to the phony "I'm just saying this for your own good." "Truth" can be a vicious weapon when used in the service of hostility, less easily brushed off than falsehood.

Most people are not accustomed to others' being real in relationship to them and often do not know how to respond. Being confused, many respond with withdrawal or hostility. Without the strength to know that "You Are Not the Target" (Huxley) of such negative emotions, you may withdraw or feel great personal hurt at the response of others to your openness. We all wish for the event of being drawn out by another and for the interest and attention of another's eyes turned solely upon us. Yet we all share in the fear of being the one to reach out to make contact with others by sharing the feelings and thoughts that we have toward another.

Many altruistic persons will allow themselves to express only the good, only the positive, only the acceptable parts of themselves. It is thought by many that to be Christian is to be good, kind, and virtuous. To be angry, to be resentful, or to be anxious or depressed in relationship to another is a sinful or an un-Christian attitude. These negative emotions are rarely shared, for they are considered unworthy and unacceptable. The end result of many of these common attitudes is that people tend to deny large parts of their experience as being valued or acceptable parts of themselves. These parts are then largely unshared. They are very rarely exposed and understood by another. We do not, however, advocate the "dumping" of neurotically based, overprinted, or displaced feelings on another, who would then be a scapegoat.

## Feelings Do Not Equal Behavior

For many reasons, we often do not express or share the strong positive or negative feelings we have toward others with those others. One of the reasons is that we expect that to have or express a strong feeling means we have to act on it further. If we are sexually attracted toward someone, we often fear that to reveal the feeling means that we will have to follow through. Or worse, we fear that to have a strong sexual feeling or a strong feeling of attraction toward another will be seen as a proposition if expressed to that other. We fear being misunderstood. These fears represent blocks to the formation of intimate bonds with others. It is important, at times, to take the risk of being misunderstood.

## Sharing versus Imposing

On the other end of the spectrum is the person who shares too much, who cannot sense when sharing becomes imposing. Everyone has a neighbor who tells everything, who lets it all hang out, constantly, nonstop. She tells you about the cute birthmark underneath her left breast, about the shortness of her husband's penis, of the argument she and her husband had last night, about the strange color of her son's urine after he eats carrots, about her latest symptoms that portend a venereal disease, about her emotional distress at the latest plight of the lead's niece on "As the World Turns." All this and you just moved in! You had expressed no initial interest in her plight, nor did you particularly want to hear all the things that she had to say.

Why isn't this neighbor a true intimate? Her ability to "share" is pronounced. She shares everything. How can anyone be more intimate? Yet the quality of her transactions is far from being intimate. The reasons are several. For one, the motives of the true intimate in sharing thoughts and feelings are the need to be understood and to give a gift of oneself to the other. The neighbor is neither seeking understanding nor giving a gift of herself. She wants a sympathetic ear, but not a relationship. She is not giving a gift of herself; she is imposing herself. She wants a listener, not a confidante. She is oblivious to the needs of the listener. Another element lacking in her relationship to you is that there is no desire for reciprocity. She is not really interested in your experience or your concerns, except insofar as necessary to keep you listening to her. Nor is she really telling everything. She tells a lot of information and many things about her life, but she never says anything about her feelings toward you in your relationship. Reflections on the nature and quality of your relationship with her are strangely lacking. Your neighbor, rather than being super-intimate, as it might at first appear, is not capable of real intimacy. Her intimacies are all second-hand, are all from the past, or from outside your relationship. Her inability to be intimate with others drives her to share those frustrations with you in an attempt to be close and receive from you the intimacy she is not capable of getting elsewhere. She shares her frustrations about her friends with you, however, not with them. And she will share her frustrations about you with someone else. She will invariably avoid real intimacy. She is a bore, not an intimate. Your best recourse in this situation is to be intimate with her in an attempt to elicit real intimacy from her. That is, you could tell her that you are terribly bored (given that you really are) and that you don't hear her being interested in you, nor do you hear her sharing any of her feelings about you.

### Instant Intimacy

Many sorts of contemporary experiences provide partial or pseudo-intimacy. One of the most obvious symbols of the intimacy vacuum felt today is the growth of the encounter movement. People flock to encounter groups, Gestalt groups, touchie-feelies, nude marathons, massage weekends. Human growth institutes are emerging like mushrooms after the rain. Humanistic psychology has multiplied its adherents. Sensitivity training is sought by IBM executives. A need is being filled in these settings that is not being met at home, in the family, within the context of friendships, or within the confines of normal everyday life. The need is for intimacy, both physical and emotional. There is total sharing, total revelation, feeling high by feeling whole or by being felt. Experiencing ourselves in bits and pieces, presenting different parts of ourselves to different people, we are fragmented by the way that we are known, by the way we present ourselves. Being more fully revealed, more totally exposed, and sharing the normally hidden, we feel whole, high, and freed. People leave their encounter experiences on a high that they ride back into the ordinary mundane world. For a time, they are bright lights in the grey nether world of everyday life. But soon the light dims; the rewards for revelation do not exist in the same way here. The risks are greater, the hurts more frequent. The total sharing of the encounter is often abandoned. Disillusioned, the encounter buff may cease to change that which is around him, cease to try being fully revealed, and cease to share in great depth. Instead, he looks forward to his next encounter weekend for an "intimacy fix." A habit is easily formed. Irvin Yalom's research on group therapies and encounter groups points out that outcomes are as varied as philosophies of movements and styles of leadership. Those groups with the most "charismatic" leaders (especially when assaultive and intrusive), regardless of orientation, though sometimes leading to an immediate "high" in their participants, have the worst long-term results as well as the most casualties. A shy but successful student at a small private university had a powerful and exhilarating experience of intimacy at an encounter weekend. Impulsively, he transferred to a large, prestigious state university. But students there were not as kind, as open as in the group. His isolation was greater than ever. He wound up on a psychiatric ward.

In closing, of all the characteristics of strength described, perhaps the most fundamental is that of being truly close to another human being, of being capable of commitment, of vulnerability, of openness, of valuing others, and of allowing oneself to be valued.

# 5

# SEX

Only one chapter on sex? What can we say here to engage the prospective reader who opens the book to this page first? Hasn't it all been said? The sequels to popular books on sex are coming out with new sequels. It's getting so that we think we know more than we ever wanted to know about sex. We've stopped asking.

The strong are *not* those with all the answers about sex. They must continue to struggle with the issues. There is no single sexual or life style among those of strength; they may be faithfully married, unmarried, or divorced, living communally, or meaningfully involved with a homosexual partner. In spite of this vagueness, reflected in the uprooting of social norms, in the shifts in definitions of sexual psychopathology (for example, the American Psychiatric Association just removed homosexuality from its diagnostic list of mental disorders), and in our own uncertainties, we do feel clear about four attributes of the strong in their sexuality. He (or she) avoids the use of sex for nonsexual motives—control, power, dependency, self-reassurance, or as a mere antidote to loneliness. He has the capability of combining sex with love and of sustaining sexual relatedness with a given partner. He does not kid himself about what he is doing; he is aware of his drives, takes into account his principles, and is aware of social pressures. Finally, he is in control; he chooses; he runs his sex life—it doesn't run him.

## The Continuous Committed Relationship

Just as sexual attraction can evoke affectionate feelings, so do affectionate feelings sustain sexual interest. The grand passion that does not entail friendship and intimacy as already described peters out. Sexual surveys point out how many older couples maintain active sexual lives into the seventies and eighties. Are not they likely the ones to have sustained tenderness? Certainly they have proved commitment to one another. (We define commitment as a pledge not to reject unless taken advantage of and, as a corollary, not to provoke being exploited.)

Commitment implies the ability to resolve conflict. No long-term, intimate relationship can be hassle-free. Making up in bed is not the answer. That skirts the issue. Good sex is a result of harmony, not a way to find it. Often the development of sexual difficulties such as orgastic failure, impotence, or premature ejaculation can be regarded as a sensitive indicator of something awry in the relationship. In other cases, "good sex" can be used, at least for a while, to "paper over" important issues that need to be resolved.

Uncle Tom boasted, "Your Aunt Jane and I haven't had a fight in our eighteen wonderful years of marriage." A little later in the evening, he went to bed drunk in his separate bedroom.

A psychologist sought couple therapy for himself and his wife because he had lost his sexual desire for her, which he attributed to her being fat. Until recently, actually, in spite of her plumpness, sex had been frequent and "great." Soon it became apparent that he had never told her of his disappointment in her overly submissive behavior, her gluttony, or about his own extramarital affairs, his homosexual fantasies. She had not revealed her sadness, her wish to be a more autonomous person, her rage at being analyzed rather than related to. Sex was the last to go.

The dilemmas presented by the fact of attraction to another and, ever more nowadays, by the possibility of acting upon it, are inevitable. Why do so many self-aware and unconstricted individuals, despite its delights and rewards, in their strength eschew the ongoing affair outside of marriage? This decision may not have come about easily. It frequently is the result of bad personal experiences. There is enormous difficulty in carrying on a affair while trying to maintain continuing intimacy with another. Secrecy breeds alienation; while frankness about outside affairs (most especially those ongoing and meaningful) can breed hurt and resentment.

As George Bach points out, conflicts and assertive behavior are intrinsic to intimacy and to the continued expression of love and sexuality together. You need to share anger when feeling anger, sexuality when feeling sexual. To try to be turned on while actually angry is either dishonest or the result of dissociation of sexuality from tenderness.

### The Ongoing Affair

As Morton Hunt states in *The Affair*, "The myth is monogamy. The fact is frequently polygamy. Our cultural heritage is thus schizoid. It offers us an approved model of marriage which, for all its values and its beauty, is suited to the needs and emotional abilities of only some—perhaps a minority—of us; it simultaneously offers a deviant, disapproved model which, for all its disadvantages, is suited to the needs and emotional abilities of the rest—perhaps even a majority—of us."

I (GFS) was deeply impressed by the answer Sally gave me when I asked her about her remarkable apparent ability to tolerate her lover's open affair with Grace. Sally said, "What matters to me is the quality of Bob's relationship to me. That hasn't changed either personally or sexually, so why should I be jealous?" Sadly, however, it took only a few more months for that quality to change and for Sally to leave. Bob simply could not maintain depth in two relationships. On the other hand, when I inquired of my Indian host, a professor of traditional medicine, if he felt able to maintain an equal love for his two wives (who happen to be sisters), with each of whom he has two children, he replied confidently, "Yes." Is the difference due to cultural acceptance? Probably it is more the result of the fact of all living together and sharing and of the harmonious relationship between the two women.

Jerry, in his cups one evening, told of his several affairs over the past few years. Unexpectedly he revealed: "I've given up on these long-term affairs. Do you know why? I'll tell you. It got so that even when I was with my wife I would be thinking about Nancy, planning when we could get together. I was never all there with my wife any more. I kidded myself that I could keep my relationships separate, but I had to face the fact finally that I couldn't. So now when I find myself continually longing for some woman, I take that energy and make things more exciting with my wife. I buy her some flowers, we have a fight and clear the air, or we spend more time together. That doesn't mean I wouldn't be tempted to have an occasional fling, but I have given up on the ongoing affair."

Obviously, our points here are not based on moral considerations or even especially on theoretical ones. We can conceive of simultaneous ongoing, nondestructive sexual relationships among the strong (spouses and lovers); pragmatically, we simply haven't observed it. Your significant relationships are significant by virtue of the fact that they touch on a vast portion of your experience, thus providing a subjective sense of wholeness and integration. To the extent that hiding and deceit remove areas of your experience from the significant other, that relationship becomes less intimate and less wholesome. A continuing affair, occupying attention, emotion, time, and requiring hiding, can only take away from a significant and primary intimate relationship. The more time, energy, and attention directed away from the primary relationship, the less viable and sustaining that relationship becomes.

## SEX WITHOUT LOVE

### Infatuation

Infatuation is not love; it may or may not lead to love. Being "head over heels" implies a projection of an ego-ideal on another. (Freud suggested that this sort of love-object represents the actual self or wished-for self and thus has strong elements of narcissism.) The truly loved is known and valued for what he or she actually is. Faults are recognized and accepted; there is no glossing over them or unrealistic belief in the ability to change them. Changes in physical attractiveness due to age or misfortune do not alter love. Perhaps one may be less likely to fall in love with a deformed person; one does not stop loving someone scarred in an accident, developing crow's feet or graying hair. (This is not to say that respect cannot be lost for someone who lacks pride in appearance, who lets himself become slovenly or obese; respect is a prerequisite for love.)

Most continuous relationships cannot compete with the excitement of a new affair. There is novelty to what is said, to what happens in bed. Day-to-day realities are not faced together. You may not see her putting on her make-up or carrying out the garbage.

### The Casual Affair

If the new affair does not become a preoccupation, an obsession, or result in the development of a pejorative attitude to the more mundane and realistic primary relationship, it may offer little danger to the primary commitment. Yet, is it fair to the "third party?" Is he or she also just out for sex and fun? Is exploitation involved? Does dishonesty cloud both relationships?

The Robinsons, married several years, have jobs that keep them apart several days a month. Both Louis and Jennifer had had brief affairs, although neither had directly admitted it to the other. Finally, the strain of the secret was too great; an agonizing confession and reappraisal of the relationship ensued. Although both had harbored fears to the contrary, it became clear that they both very much wanted to continue a life together. On the other hand, brief interludes were both convenient and easy for each. Neither felt the heavy hand of conventional moral restraint on acting out sexual feelings. Having fully confronted their jealousy and their fears of being abandoned, they found a new freedom to accept the casual affairs of the other. Jennifer reported, "We decided to avoid continuing affairs as being far too threatening. In fact, I have even broken off a relationship that might compete for too much of my time. We are also working much harder to make the time we have together quality time."

Jay and Mae Ziskin report in *The Extra-Marital Sex Contract* that in interviewing 124 couples who had mutually entered a contract agreeing to engage in extramarital sex, dating, separate vacations, three-day weekends with others, casual affairs were found to be workable, but that "It is almost always a condition of the co-marital sex contract that deep relationships are to be avoided under this concept. It is falling in love, not going to bed, that constitutes infidelity." Among these couples, clandestine affairs were almost invariably found to be dangerous.

The Ziskins concluded from their observations that several conditions were necessary for nondestructive and, according to their interviewees, healthful extramarital sex: open and frequent communication about the contract both before and during; acceptance of the natural feelings of each other for variety, stimulation, and new experiences; the willingness to have a trial run and to carefully evaluate the experience; and a clear set of groundrules about time, place, extent of disclosures about activities, and people (usually friends) who are to be off limits.

Of particular interest to us was an observation about these couples: "They seem to possess a more than average amount of that quality often referred to as 'ego strength.' " They were sure of themselves, charted their own courses, yet not at the expense of the feelings of others, including the "affairee."

In more troubled marriages, the affair, though not healthy in the sense that it is an integrative force in the marriage or a mature decision mutually agreed upon, may serve some good. It may serve as a clear index that there is real trouble in the marriage, that the ability of the two persons to be mutually rewarding and supplying of affection and support to one another has diminished to such a point that one of the persons turns elsewhere for his or her affection and loving. Although this action is an avoidance of conflict and reflects an inability to confront troubled areas in a marriage, it may indicate that necessary satisfaction and conflict resolution are lacking in the marriage. If the resentment and bitterness that may have built up are not yet too great, intervention at this point by the knowledge of and the confrontation with the meaning of an affair may help the marriage to grow rather than wilt.

## Nonsexual Motivations for Sex

We have stated that the strong tend not to kid themselves, about sex or other considerations. If they seek sex because of horniness, they can admit it. More importantly, they do not disguise other strivings as sexual. We already have described the Don Juan and the femme fatale who seduce to conquer, the manipulator who uses sexuality in the service of control, and the emotional isolate who seeks fleeting contact through impersonal sex. The list could go on. Aggressive motivations readily fuse with sexual, the most obvious and ultimate form of which is rape. Yet more subtle forms of hostile sex abound both in the forms of masochistic submission and sadistic exploitation.

Susan, a stunningly attractive blonde, reported to her psychiatrist shortly after her admission to the hospital for an acute manic psychosis, that she had been seduced by her college counselor. The newly trained counselor, a product of a sexually restrictive cultural tradition, had recently been "liberated" by his experience in the encounter and Gestalt movements. He perceived correctly that Susan had been sadly neglected by her wealthy, social parents. He felt she needed compensation through being held and touched for several hours a week. Susan never was literally seduced. What the counselor courageously became able to face was that in his own unmet needs for tenderness and sexuality he had exploited his client.

In contrast stands the middle-aged ex-priest who, taking a course in massage techniques, openly admitted, "I like to touch bodies." How refreshing!

A particularly malignant and often well-hidden nonsexual motivation that can seriously impair sexual fulfillment, one that is becoming far more prevalent in contemporary times, is the need to perform, to achieve. Those couples not reaching simultaneous orgasm 85.6 percent of the time may consider themselves inadequate, failures. Although sexual fulfillment in life is a legitimate expectation, it can easily become a demand. The "new impotence" arises not from the frigidity of the spouse but from fears of being unable to keep up with her. Skilled sexual therapists achieve good results not so much through training in technique as by fostering harmony within the relationship and in removing sex from the arenas of competition, who is getting what from whom, and from "objective" standards of "competence."

## LOVE WITHOUT SEX

Were Plato's feelings for his students really platonic? Certainly his mentor, Socrates, freely acknowledged his sexual attraction to Alcibiades. What Plato seemed to say more than to deny the physical was rather to idealize the spiritual aspect of relatedness. Emotional closeness is often followed by sexual feelings and attraction. The border is not as distinct as many would like to think. To avoid sexual feelings some avoid closeness. Is it not better to allow the closeness and deal appropriately with whatever attraction may ensue?

Though the strong person may well be more able to love in the absence of sexual feelings, to be better able to differentiate affectionate and genital strivings, he also is less likely to be threatened or thwarted by the presence of sexual reactions. We have already pointed out how strength is manifest in the ability to differentiate between thought or impulse and action. Certainly, those choosing a celibate life style for religious or spiritual reasons need not be unloving persons. They are in danger only when they deny their sexuality to themselves. A young priest related, "Many upon many of my priest friends have innocently undertaken the role of counselor and spiritual advisor to nuns in a nearby convent only to end up in what amounts to a pattern of dating under another name. More than several asked me, 'Why in God's name did we end up in bed? I had no intention. . . .' "

## CONTROL

As we have just illustrated, sexual feelings need not be feared when their expression is channeled through rationality that takes into account the effects of sexual behavior on the sexual partners, other significant persons in each other's lives, and on one's self-esteem and view of himself.

In contrast, an element of "letting go," of spontaneity, of voluntary noncontrol is essential for the fullness of sexual expressivity and sensual enjoyment. In psychoanalytic terms, the ego builds a playpen in which the id can romp, or in transactional analysis terms, the adult defines the area wherein the child can freely and safely play.

For many, it is almost as difficult to let go of control as it is to express negative feelings. It is thus a mark of strength that you are able to "let go." Orgasm is in some ways a primitive and total loss of control ("little death," in a French expression), a brief state of pure "id" or instinct, if you will. To be sexually exposed, out of control in a sense, to let go emotionally and to allow free expression of love and affection while participating in lovemaking are difficult and, for the frigid, impossible. Stronger persons experience the full range of their feelings, secure in their ability to regain control. "Letting go" implies a choice to abandon control temporarily. It is as restricting to feel one must only express sexuality by means of genital contact with the male in the active role as it is to feel one must be a sexual athlete practicing each of the 105 positions of the most recent sex manual.

## SEXUAL STYLES

Life style has much to do with sexuality, as does sexual preference with life style. Formerly secretive pairings, particularly the homosexual choice, are coming out of the closet. The straight have no monopoly upon strength. Indeed, unconventional life and sexual styles may require special fortitude to be maintained honestly in the face of social disapproval. The issue is not the partner or partners *per se,* but the quality and harmony of sexuality in the service of inner mastery and interpersonal fulfillment.

As men and women become more aware of their emotional and sexual selves, as they discover new alternatives, and as they free themselves of restrictive cultural sanctions, new sexual styles may emerge. Group living and sexuality is one possibility. However, if two people cannot make it consistently with one another, it seems unlikely they will be able to make it with a group. If someone cannot love, he or she will fail with a lover or with lovers. Until problems are solved in relationship to individuals, there is faint hope that group marriages would fare any better than pairings. Multiple, shallow relationships are no substitute for deep and committed ones. However, we do not feel that the nuclear family is necessarily God-given. It is perhaps among the strong, capable of intimacy with individuals and with groups, not bound to traditional modes, that new, workable life styles may be developed for others to follow. Indeed, recapturing some of the benefits of the old, extended family in new ways has much appeal. Certainly, the kibbutz, with its combination of pairings and groupings, with individuality and collectivism, with both the nuclear and extended family, is one such alternative.

## FANTASY

Sexual fantasies are universal. They may represent what we do or what we should like to do. They may tell symbolic stories. They may fulfill unconscious needs. They may be acceptable or alien. It is not uncommon that one's fantasies may become preoccupying, taking attention away from a current involvement, making one's present existence look mundane and uninteresting (even if it is relatively good). When fantasizing occurs chronically and everyday life becomes bleak in comparison, it may be necessary to reassess your current life. One way to lay a fantasy to rest is to make it a reality, to give it a trial run. This acting-out runs the danger, however, of being rewarding, thereby inviting compulsive repetition. If you fantasize special kinds of sex, and this makes current sex tame by comparison, it may be helpful to try it. By bringing a fantasy down to reality, you can then make realistic judgments about its virtues and drawbacks. You can then either more easily give up the fantasy or change your reality.

In conclusion, the sexual life of a strong person cannot be rigidly characterized any more than can any other aspect of his or her life. He or she does find sexuality most satisfying in the service of relatedness and intimacy, does not deny his or her sensuality, does not combine sexual and nonsexual motives, and is not driven by sexual aims to the exclusion of his or her own ethical and rational considerations.

# 6
# AGGRESSION

Is the strong person aggressive? Is the aggressive person strong? Do the strong turn the other cheek?

A quiet young man described by neighbors and acquaintances as polite, studious, and kindly shoots down passers-by randomly from a tower. A former Golden Gloves welterweight champ allows his boss to steal his ideas without protest. The young woman next door, whose husband always seemed so solicitous of her, appears one day with a black eye, and her "doorknob" story sounds phony. When is aggression appropriate? How does inappropriate, apparently inexplicable aggression occur?

## THEORIES OF AGGRESSION

First, what is aggression? The word's Latin root simply means "to move toward." Aggression, thus, can refer both to assertive motivations and to hostile ones. In the assertive sense come such behaviors as standing up for your rights, striving for competence, ambitiousness, living up to potentialities, getting your due. Hostility has to do with anger and the wish to harm. Aggression in its service is the act of inflicting hurt, in its ultimate form violence. We shall differentiate the assertive from the hostile, but for purposes of simplicity and common usage shall reserve the term "aggression" for hostile behaviors.

There are three basic categories of aggression theory. First are instinctual theories that place aggression as an innate component of man's biological, inherited make-up. Freud based sexuality and affection in a biological life force (Eros) and aggression in a death instinct (Thantos). Ethnologists like Konrad Lorenz analogize to humans from the prevalence of intraspecies aggression among other species, which fight to defend territory, to compete for mates, and to establish dominance. In the second category fall the frustration-aggression hypotheses. When strivings to meet needs and wants are blocked, frustration and anger, which can lead to attack, ensue. Finally, social learning theories emphasize example and early experience. If your parents, your favorite TV hero, or your country fight to resolve conflict or achieve aims, that's how you learn to do so, too. No theory is necessarily exclusive of others.

Some see man as intrinsically bad, having to overcome base instincts or Original Sin through socialization, indoctrination, fear, or coercion. Freud saw love more as an antidote to hate than as a preventive of it. He feared that the more civilization suppressed man's aggressive drives, the greater the likelihood of their outbreak in ever more destructive wars. Fundamentalist preachers believe they must keep parishioners in line through fear of hellfire. On the other side, some—such as the nineteenth-century anarchists and some of the new libertarians—see man as intrinsically good, needing only to be unfettered from the shackles of oppressive society. We take neither position. Man has the potentiality for the greatest good—altruism and selflessness, lacking in lower animals (but perhaps manifested by the monkey sacrificing itself by leading a predator away from the troop); and the greatest evil—sadism, torture, genocide, the indiscriminate destruction of war. Man's aggressive potentialities clearly have biological roots. Their expression has to do with developmental and social forces.

## PRIMARY AND SECONDARY AGGRESSION

When nothing works, you get angry. What then? The anger can be repressed (shoved out of consciousness); defended against by various self-deceiving maneuvers such as projection (thinking it's really the other who is hostile), displacement (kicking the dog), or sublimation (handled in acceptable but indirect ways such as working out with a punching bag); or it can be directly expressed. If the expression is in direct response to and proportional with the frustrating or provoking situation, the response can be termed *primary aggression*. Such aggression, if complete, permanently reduces tension. "Getting it off your chest" or "out of your system" prevents repression and build-up of hostile impulses.

Strength may be involved in the ability to express the primary, appropriate form of aggression, which can, of course, vary in intensity from mild annoyance to killing in the service of self-defense, depending upon the provocation. If someone at work consistently uses his coffee cup, leaving it unwashed in the sink, the strong person is likely to take a stand. If a rapist, after stabbing her husband, is coming at her with switchblade drawn, the strong woman may well furtively grasp the butcher knife lying on the nearby counter. Yet sometimes even primary aggression needs to be channeled or controlled. However appropriate your anger at an unreasonable boss, thought may be wise before reacting to him. Decision must be made about the appropriateness of hostile feelings in terms of whether they really are proportional to the frustration (primary), and choices then made about modes of expressing aggression.

*Secondary aggression* is not based on, though perhaps is precipitated by, current provocation or frustration. It is unprovoked or out of proportion. Its roots lie in unrelieved old frustrations dealt with chronically through repression. Yet secondary aggression arises not merely from a "storehouse" of hostility, for if that were true, chip-on-the-shoulder behaviors should eventually deplete the storehouse. Such is not the case. Unprovoked and out-of-proportion hostile and violent behavior tends to occur over and over. It may serve some defensive purpose as anxiety relief; yet expression of inappropriate resentments creates new frustrations. Like the resolution of other neurotic patterns, its solution lies in discovering the conflicts underlying the behavior and working them through in the context of present relationships. Those whose secondary aggression is out of control must be controlled by society.

## PREVENTING AGGRESSION

The following diagram illustrates the points made and provides a model for our subsequent discussion of prevention of inappropriate aggression. Numbers refer to points at which effective modes of intervention can be instituted. (We shall not discuss intervention at point 5—repression and defense—because, as mentioned, such is generally a matter for psychotherapeutic uncovering.) Points 6 and 7—actual aggression—will be discussed primarily in terms of handling the aggression of others. Strategies for healthy control of aggression can be undertaken at any point along the chain of events. The earlier the intervention, the easier. The strong are most likely to have the widest repertoire of such strategies; as your repertoire broadens, you become stronger.

Figure 1

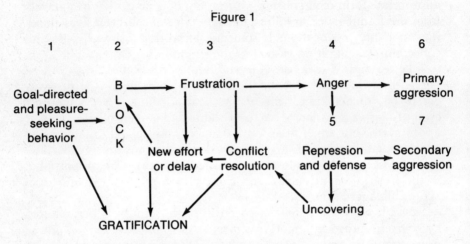

### Interventions at the Goal-Setting Stage—1

*Too many goals.* Hopes, wishes, fantasies, desires, and expectations of others and of ourselves are all goals. The more goals and expectations you have, the more probable it is that you will encounter blocks to your goals in life. Many of us have far too many unrealistic expectations of others, of how situations ought to be, of how we ought to behave, or of how others ought to behave, thus setting ourselves up for frustration and anger.

I (GFS) find I have a narrow range between feeling bored and feeling overwhelmed. Recently, an able prospective assistant hesitated to accept the job because she thought what I was trying to do alone was too much for two. I now have two scientific papers due, besides a new psychiatric training program and a new treatment program for criminal offenders, both getting underway. Though I enjoy each task, the combination is too much. I'm feeling both angry and sorry for myself, yet I've done it to myself.

*Goals unset.* Frustration can arise not only from goals unmet, but from goals unset. Overstimulation, continual change, and too many options are stressful, but so are understimulation, monotony, and boredom. We feel that lack of fulfillment of at least some of one's intrinsic potentialities, which may not even be consciously perceived, is frustrating. The highly coordinated person who never engages in sports, the person with the lovely voice who never sings, the intelligent person who never thinks, are all frustrated at some level. Freud thought that the organism always sought reduction of tension. This clearly is not the case. Understimulated animals and people seek stimulation. Sensory deprivation is highly stressful. Those who antici- pate defeat and frustration, particularly, are those who avoid setting goals.

*Overly high expectations.* Even realistic goals meet with impediments leading to frustration of various degrees. Unrealistic goals are even worse. Many people add to their frustration because they basically do not accept themselves for having negative emotions. "What a stupid thing to feel!" "That feeling is completely irrational." "I shouldn't feel that." Having an image of or goal for themselves as persons whose feelings "should" be rational, they are doomed to perpetual failure of their self-expectations. Thus, each negative emotion from other causes is compounded by a person's own lack of acceptance of negative emotions within himself. Some frustrations are inevitable. Such acceptance actually leads to greater probability of eventual goal achievement.

There is a balance between having hopes and expectations that allow you to move toward rewarding and worthwhile goals and having so many unrealistic and unneeded goals and expectations that you are continually frustrated and debilitated. Jackie finally gave up beating her head against the wall trying to be a research chemist and took up nursing, even though it was not the "liberated" thing to do. She has since made up with her boyfriend, has upped her grade point average, and even has some time for relaxation.

*Having the wrong goals.* Many of us feel that we have to be very special and do lofty and worthwhile things to earn love from others. Other times we just don't know where we are heading or why. A beloved and gifted colleague and co-worker struggled long and hard to obtain his Ph.D. in psychology relatively late in life. We were all proud of him when it was finally awarded. We were at first shocked and taken aback when he and his family moved to a small distant town, where he spent much time in meditation and in restoring an old Victorian house while supporting himself and family by working as a school janitor. Our first reaction was to think he had flipped. Only when he returned on a visit did we realize what true peace he had achieved. He no longer chain-smoked; the fine tremor in his hands was gone. Yet, could he have changed his life style and established revised goals without having first met his goal of getting a doctorate?

### *Interventions at the Barriers to Goals—2*

Some barriers to goals are insurmountable and need to be accepted as such. Some are psychological products of one's own negative self-image ("I can't do it.") and need to be surmounted through personal growth. Some are real, but can be confronted with greater energy. Some are temporary, and waiting needs to be accepted as the most appropriate solution. The number of life skills you acquire increases your ability to circumvent barriers, avoid frustration, and thus become destructively aggressive less often.

Kay, sportscar-loving but not wealthy, became frustrated by the inconvenience, poor workmanship, and expense involved in the maintenance of her finicky Italian machine. She took a mechanic's course at a local community college and now not only lacks those frustrations, but has the fun of her newfound hobby of working on her own and friends' cars.

### *Interventions When You Are Frustrated—3*

Our society socializes people to make two different, both potentially harmful responses: on the one hand, to repress negative feelings as much as possible (be a nice guy) and, on the other hand, to resort to aggression early in the hierarchy of responses when frustrated (be a hard guy). Certainly, we know that some soldiers in Vietnam learned that "wasting gooks" was the simplest response and had a hard time with their resultant guilt and lack of control of aggression as returned veterans. As pointed out, these aggressive propensities are aggravated by unresolved feelings resulting from prior repression. The strong tend to have a variety of alternatives to both repression and explosiveness in their handling of frustration.

*Monitoring stress.* Stress of various kinds is directly related to frustration. The greater the variety and intensity of stresses, physical and psychological, at any given time, the greater the likelihood of frustration in trying to cope with them. At some point, any individual's coping mechanisms can break down, resulting in a variety of symptoms—anxiety, hostility, physical illness, or aggressive behaviors.

Thomas Holmes, for example, has reported research which related life changes to physical and mental health. It is possible to assess quantitatively the number of life changes that one undergoes during a period of time. Some items on his list of significant changes include marriage, death of spouse, a mortgage over $10,000, buying a new car, moving into a new house, being promoted, and so on. Each item is assigned a point value based on the ratings of a large group of people. *Any change,* it was discovered, added stress to life even if it was one that is perceived as positive, such as moving into a new house or getting a promotion. The total number of points on the change-of-life scale was directly correlated with the number of physical and mental problems in a person's life.

*Finishing uncompleted tasks.* An old Gestalt notion states that people seek closure for tasks and that there is energy still bound up with uncompleted tasks. The more uncompleted tasks or goal-directed behaviors in our lives at one time, the less energy available for coping with current life situations, the less energy available to cope with current frustrations; hence, there is greater propensity for aggression, violent outbursts, depressions, and secondary aggression.

The problem is growing. Multiplicity of life changes and overstimulation are rapidly becoming major problems for the average citizen. Alvin Toffler makes the point that "there are finite boundaries; we are not infinitely resilient. Each orientation response, each adaptive reaction enacts a price, wearing down the body's machinery bit by minute bit, until perceptible tissue damage results . . . there are discoverable limits to the amount of change that the human organism can absorb, and . . . by endlessly accelerating change without first determining these limits, we may submit masses of men to demands they simply cannot tolerate."

The simple device of listing all of the uncompleted tasks in current life and then systematically checking them off the list by completing the tasks often has the consequence of dramatically changing your mood, of lifting a burden. Uncompleted tasks may be as simple as having yet to mail a letter, to go to the store, to make the bed, to wash the windows, to fix that annoying noise in the car, or to file a report due at work, to need to make up with a friend, or even to have to make a list in order to get the things done. The dramatic feeling change often accompanying the completion of these seemingly simple and inconsequential tasks is the result of the release for full use in the present of energy currently being used up attending to the incompletion of the tasks. Sometimes a seemingly depressed client is not suffering from the classical neurosis or physical depletion, but merely from too many things hanging. Closure cures. The preoccupied person is easily recognizable because he seems distant, appears to be in another world. He is dealing with uncompleted tasks and unfulfilled dreams, wishes, and fantasies. The person who is entirely present when he is with you has mastered his past and current personal life tasks and current environmental demands and so can attend completely.

*Recognizing the frustration.* A tax consultant, in treatment because of unexplained angry outbursts, never knew when he was frustrated or upset until he exploded. It helps to be aware of the sensations associated with anger and frustration. Many act without being fully aware of their feelings or without being able to verbalize what feelings underlie their actions. Awareness of frustration is necessary for conceptual control of the negative emotions associated. The conversion of emotion from a percept (subjective sensation or feeling) to a concept (an idea expressed by language symbols) itself is a step toward control and mastery (and is one of the important elements of psychotherapy).

*Sublimation.* Upon awareness of anger, many choose sublimation as a means of handling that feeling. In sublimation, unlike other defenses, the wish or drive is expressed rather than repressed, but its aim or object altered to be more acceptable to self or others. A choice can be made to discharge emotion through action, such as through sports, debate, nonviolent protest, competition, and similar means. Because it is a constructive way of discharging negative emotion, sublimation is a particularly useful way of channeling impulses to aggression. It is not the ideal way of handling negative emotions, however, for it often does not allow full discharge of the feelings involved or resolution of the underlying conflict. Working out on a punching bag after a fight with one's wife may be more appropriate than beating her, but may not in the long run prevent further frustration and aggression. A strong person can sublimate, but more often attempts directly to discharge his feeling in adaptive ways.

*Passive, aggressive, and assertive responses.* A situation calling for constructive assertion may be completely avoided because of the associations that aggressiveness has with assertion. The result may be a passive Milquetoast who never stands up for his rights and lets others walk all over him. This passive person then, building up storehouses of hostility, may be predisposed to various forms of secondary aggression.

Anyone's own reaction to frustration can occur in three modes. One may be aggressive and cruel, lashing out, attacking others, inflicting pain, making others take the toll for his negative feelings. In the passive response, one swallows his frustration and forsakes his goals or hopes and suffers in silence or disguises the expression of rage through passive resistance and obstruction ("I'm too tired to go to the movie"). Or, in the masochistic vein, one becomes the victim of his own aggression, a mechanism involved in depressive illness. (Of course, the masochist or martyr also expresses his hostility by trying to provoke guilt in others.) In the short run, the passive person takes a toll from himself, giving up his own goals and desires rather than evoking conflict or, as he sees it, imposing on others. The assertive person is not apt to deny himself, his goals, his feelings, or his wants in a frustrating situation, but rather assesses his personal rights and tries to find a way to meet his needs without inflicting unnecessary hurt on either himself or others.

Let's, for example, role-play an ordinary dining-out situation. I, the passive guy, order a rare steak. The waitress brings me one well-done. I am in a dilemma. Shall I, fearful of a hassle, swallow the steak along with my frustration and an Alka Seltzer? I decide upon the alternative. More truthfully, my wife decides for me: "Send that miserable excuse for a steak back to the cook. At these prices! The nerve!"

Having rehearsed my line, I beckon the waitress: "Please, Miss, is there any way that I could possibly have a steak a little less brown in the center?"

Wife: "Like bleeding!"

Husband, recovering the ball: "I . . . I'm not blaming you, Miss, I know these things happen." So the weak man goes on, apologizing, agonizing.

Now, in the same situation, I assume the role of a stronger person—no incensed berating, no well-turned phrase demanding better service, and no indigestion. Keeping in mind the feelings of the waitress, and clearly cognizant of her tired feet, I explain: "I won't enjoy my dinner unless I get the blood-rare steak I ordered."

The virtue of assertiveness is the avoidance of both direct aggression and the subtle toll taken by repression. Strategies of assertiveness are rarely modeled by parents, rarely talked about in books on aggression, and are not likely to have been learned through a course other than that of a life sensitively lived in relationship to others and through many personal conflicts.

*Demanding to be divined.* If you want someone to know what you're feeling, tell him. When our own feelings are so strong, so clearly felt, it is easy to assume that any sensitive person can pick up our feelings. If he doesn't, then it often seems that he must not care. Why else would he ignore our feelings? But others are not mind-readers. More than one interpersonal disaster has begun when one of the parties has demanded to be divined.

So often the weaker hint about their feelings, both wanting to reveal and to hide at the same time, never daring to take responsibility for explicitness. They want to be sure of the reaction before committing themselves to revealing. The strong decide whether to reveal or to keep hidden a feeling; they don't try to do both simultaneously.

Genevieve had had a particularly difficult day with the children. Little Bobby developed bronchitis, and there was a long wait at the pediatrician's office. Michelle, jealous over all the attention to Bobby, was bratty. Genevieve regaled Wilt with this frustration upon his return from work and made a point of how many Excedrins she had taken. She became enraged when he went on to watch Walter Cronkite instead of setting the table. She had never said, "I'm really behind with dinner. Could you help out?" No wonder Genevieve didn't have an orgasm that night.

### Intervention When Angry—4

*The pressure-cooker analogy.* "I know what happens when I bottle up my feelings—they eventually explode." Such is a not uncommon rationalization for hostile outbursts. Even when hostility is appropriate, wisdom need be exercised in its mode of expression. Outbursts of anger may release your tension, but they do not necessarily bring resolution. While meeting your need for ventilation, the needs and feelings of the person attacked can be left unconsidered. Even worse, you may so alienate the attacked person that he may not be predisposed to help you or empathize with you for the upsetting problem. Conflict resolution is then impaired rather than fostered, just as if the issue had not been dealt with at all.

*Anger as a decision to hurt.* Anger and hostility are almost always attempts to punish another person, to inflict hurt, to strike back. Thomas Gordon makes the point that when you say you are angry, it is almost never the basic, underlying feeling that is being expressed. It is almost always misleading to report merely that you are "angry" with someone. Anger is considered by Gordon to be a disguised "you message"—for example, an attempt to put the problem on the other person ("You make me mad"), to say that the other person was the cause of your feelings. Such anger is actually your attempt to punish or hurt the other person rather than a genuine attempt to communicate in such a way as to allow understanding of your feelings.

*Share, don't attack.* In actuality, the real choice being made is between sharing and attacking ("I am feeling damn jealous" versus "You goddam lecher!"), between being intimate and pursuing the goal of punishing or inflicting pain (either physical or psychological) on others. An unexplained hostile outburst is a way of punishing another.

Intimacy implies sharing fully of yourself, including the negative, demonic side. Awareness is required in order that cognitive control may be exerted over the response to the feelings. It is not generally realized that you have a choice as to how you express your negative emotions. But it is precisely at this point, between the frustration and the aggression, that choice can be exercised, where you can either share or attack, either be intimate or hostile, strong or weak.

*Anger does not dictate its expression.* It is more difficult to share than to attack because most people think that a feeling dictates its expression. A young mother of several rambunctious youngsters reported to her parent effectiveness training group: "The kids were fighting in the back of the car. I thought this was my chance to try my new skills. So I tried the suggested 'I-message'—'I get so angry, Jimmy, when you fight that I just want to hit you!' Pow! I hit him. I guess I'll never learn!"

### Intervention When Aggression Occurs—5

Developing a clear sense of responsibility for his own reactions and behavior is a device used by a strong person to handle the aggression of others and his own consequent retaliatory impulses. Knowing to whom a problem really belongs substantially reduces your own involvement in a problem not essentially yours. Obviously, anger and hostility from others elicit similar responses in ourselves. The stronger person is likely to try to help the angry person better understand the nature and sources of his own feelings; to accept blame if he is to blame and not to be inappropriately defensive; to attempt to make amends if wrong. He acknowledges the right of others to feel anger, but may confront them with their responsibility for their behavior. He does not typically escalate rage by counterattack. If violence ensues, he attempts to control and contain rather than to combat it. He always uses the least force necessary, but does not hesitate to intervene quickly before a situation gets out of hand. He tries to protect an enraged and out-of-control person from himself. Obviously, when facing the anger of a person significant to you, there is a greater need for conflict resolution; while, with a stranger, tension reduction or avoidance of further conflict may suffice. A strong person tends to be able to be hurt by those important to him, but to be less vulnerable to attacks from those he does not know or, particularly, from those he does not respect. He takes to heart legitimate criticism, but realizes that, as a strong person with definite ideas, he will inevitably offend some. He is neither insensitive nor easily devastated.

PART FOUR:

Outer Mastery

# 7

# WORK AND PLAY

Morris came in for treatment depressed, lethargic, and despairing in spite of his charming wife and delightful children. "I wasn't cut out for selling life insurance. I make good money, but I have to force myself to get out of bed in the morning when I even think about work." A major source of meaningfulness comes through what you do, through your competencies, your *outer masteries*. Robert White states, "the growth of the personality, culminating in such overall concepts as self-esteem and ego strength, can be fully understood only if we include ideas about the power to produce effects on the environment."

## Competence

To White, competence refers to both interpersonal and outer mastery: "Sense of competence signifies the degree to which a person feels able to produce desired effects upon his environment, human and inanimate—how able he feels to secure the goals that are important to him and elicit from others the behavior he desires." Competence leads to confidence and a sense of efficacy, lessens anxiety that is set off by a perception of helplessness or inadequacy, and fosters self-respect. Some psychoanalysts say the urge to mastery is an autonomous drive; others place it in the service of aggression. Ethnologists compare it with the "exploratory" or "manipulative" drives of animals. Paul McReynolds has shown, for example, that mice reared in a barren environment avoid exploration and are timid and frightened; whereas those which had repeated experiences with new "toys" and objects are bold and adventuresome in later life. At any rate, clearly effective work and play that are exploratory or leading to a sense of competence are self-fulfilling activities. In the case of play, another factor also seems present, the pleasure derived from the activity *per se*, regardless of outcome, activity that could be thus classified as "frivolous."

### An American Neurosis: Unintegrated Work

In the arena of action, strength is enhanced by finding resolution of apparent conflicts between work and play, having fun and being responsible, living fully and earning money, finding success and love. These tasks are especially difficult in America, as William Hedgepeth and Dennis Stock point out in *The Alternative*, a book on communal life:

> America is a compartmentalized land where every action, object and perception is cast by men's minds into a separate niche. Nothing is conceived to fit together. . . . The fragmented American views his job with all the relish of a zombie, sees his home life as a prison, considers culture a diversion, sex a stand-in for aggression, thinks gentleness a way of acting that brands a man a fag, and believes, deep down, that dignity essentially means the wearing of a vest. He's enamored of exactitudes, technological devices, all things vaguely scientific, total cold-eyed rationality, and those machines that help diminish human contact. For pleasure, he has learned to thrive on things that lie beyond his reach, like go-go girls he gapes at as they bump and grind securely closed in cages. He is cut off from all his senses, unaccustomed to emotions, plainly frightened of his own body, drained of the juices of humanity, ground down dull by daily living, finding comfort in his solitary boredom through his hates and prejudicial notions. God, to him is something huge and hallowed, somewhat haughty, frigid and forever personally remote. Nothing fits together; everything is either useful or it has no business being. Furthermore, with America being an outer-directed society, with emphasis on material wealth, individual success, competition and mastery over nature, it is difficult to integrate and balance inner values as a life style.

Strength is required to value your inner life, your inner feelings and needs, your interpersonal involvement, your life in the present, and to seek work in order to live rather than to live in the service of work—or, better yet, to seek life in work and work in life, trying to transcend the distinctions between work and play, between work and life.

As long as the sole reason for a job is that it provides income, security, and possible success, then synergy between work and other values is difficult or impossible. The resulting syndrome is seen in many ways: *The Man in the Grey Flannel Suit*, the bar stop before and after work, lackadaisical work performance, shoddy production, absenteeism, and lack of company loyalty. Because security was chosen over meaningful work, the manpower was available which made the Industrial Revolution possible. Many were satisfied to work at anything provided there was security and adequate wages. Other needs were suppressed in the process.

### The Great American Weekend

The great American weekend symbolizes the lack of synergy between work and play. Too many Americans work, not so much because it is rewarding and involving, but so that they can save enough money to go somewhere on the weekend, so they can have that memorable two-week package tour of the Caribbean, seven islands included. They rush to the mountains in their motor homes, only to turn on the television after chatting over burned steaks and beer with the denizens of the next motor home ten feet away. The play that is an escape from work becomes as hollow and meaningless as the work itself. Although it is often difficult, inner peace is enhanced by continually striving to find ways to bring work and play more nearly into alignment, by seeking to reduce dissonance in life.

### Humanizing Work

Strength is often found among those agents of change who attempt to humanize work situations. One way in which strong persons often have found meaning in work is to seek valued personal relationships through work. My (JAK) unassuming and quiet secretary, of South American origin, works in an office of scientifically oriented professionals. In subtle ways, she has taught them to appreciate traditions and some of the more delicate human values. Each person in the office has found a list of birthdays on his or her calendar. She asks me when to set the date for a Christmas gathering. Her influence became most visible one day when a bouquet of flowers arrived for her. It was

"National Secretaries' Week." It was bought by those who sometimes forget their own anniversaries.

The management of the Saab Automobile Works in Sweden, in consultation with its employees, is now experimenting with a team approach to assembly. Monotonous tasks can be shifted among members of the team according to their own choices and scheduling. Only the overall task is time-limited. The team produces a finished unit. It will be interesting to see whether such approaches mitigate the boredom and meaninglessness of mass-production work.

The Japanese approach to mass production has been somewhat different and perhaps is most workable in their culture. Certainly, their industrial disputes have been relatively few. Yet the new Sony plant in America is to be run on the same principles. The main effort is to make all the employees feel part of a family. Athletic, recreational, and cultural activities are brought into the plant or occur as joint ventures of co-workers during leisure. Managers are readily visible and accessible. The higher-ups know many line employees on a first-name basis. Complaints and suggestions are listened to, not just dropped in a box. Are Japanese plant managers stronger or simply wiser? Certainly, Great Britain, the industrial status of which has slipped so badly, has the opposite situation. Managers and workers tend to come from distinct cultural and educational backgrounds, have different accents, and tend to view each other as adversaries.

### Work as a Substitute for Love

A famous surgeon suffered a profound depression and ultimately committed suicide as a result of the rejection he perceived by his wife and young adult children and in the face of threats to achievement-supported self-esteem by the competition from younger surgeons trained in newer techniques. He felt that because he worked day and night, was world-renowned, and earned a great deal of money, his family should love him. They, in fact, resented him because he never gave of himself to them and never directly showed his love. A strong person does not work in order to earn the love of others. He works to meet basic needs and to gain intrinsic satisfactions. The surgeon really did care for his family. He did not know how adequately to express it. For a youth, on the other hand, to be intolerant and judgmental of such a father, who did the best he could to express his caring in the light of his own understanding arising out of his own limiting history, is a sign that the youth has not yet achieved a sense of inner peace that would allow him to be understanding rather than condemning of his parent.

It was Freud, the complex and profound psychological theoretician, who replied so simply to the query, "What is a normal person?" by answering in effect "Someone who can work and who can love."

### Radical Attempts to Integrate Life

Where the pace of change has been too slow, many people have adopted more radical attitudes in the search for living as wholly and meaningfully as possible. Drawing on personal strength and courage to be different, some have taken very clear stands in their relation to money as a symbol of success and material comfort. David Steinberg in *Working Loose*, for example, relates some of his personal decisions and reflections about money and work in his life:

> If I confuse working with making money, I'm letting other people decide when I'm working and when I'm not. When other people like my work, they buy it. Their money expresses their sense of me. But my own sense of work has no particular relationship to money or outside approval. . . . I know I'm working from the feeling I get, the work feeling, a coming alive, involvement, energy flow. Getting in tune with myself, feeling all the different parts of me coming together. Moving ahead together. . . . If I sit and perform the same job twice a minute, 120 times an hour, 5000 times a week, am I working? I can be almost asleep, repeat myself endlessly and be paid well. Or perhaps my mind will wander awake, and then it will work while my hands earn money. . . . If I have to choose between work and money, I will choose work and learn how not to need so much money. This, although I'm married and expect a baby in the next two weeks. I find that the more "family responsibility" I gain, the less I want to sacrifice myself to a need for money. I see that as I have had less and less money I have been happier with my work and with myself. I think of my relationship with my parents and resolve even more strongly to give my kids an open, loving father, even if that should mean fewer clothes and toys. . . . It's not that I have anything against money. I enjoy discovering what I can do without, but I don't enjoy being poor. It's just that when I think of what I would have to give up in order to have money I decide that it's not worth it.

In this spirit, many people, mostly young, have gone into crafts and small businesses. Attempting to integrate work and living more fully, little craft shops have begun to dot tourist centers, offering macramé, découpage, leather work, bottle-cutting, woodwork, ironwork, pottery, handmade clothes, bakery goods, health foods, paintings, driftwood objects, and endless creative and new handiworks. Art colonies and art communes scattered across the United States are becoming common. Large hardware stores and even supermarkets are beginning to carry art supplies. Much of the craft movement and the rise of communes and interest in "back-to-nature" activities is a product of what many perceive to be a loss of contact with oneself, with man's alienation from his environment, his loss of manual and physical skills, his losing touch with the ability to express himself bodily. Craftsmanship provides a sense of mastery, independence, completion, and creation. Money is sacrificed, but meaningfulness is often the profit.

One of the boldest attempts to integrate values, work, relationships, needs for community, love, and the spectrum of human needs is the commune. Comments made by commune dwellers across the country, quoted in *The Alternative*, reflect this seeking for synthesis. At "Libre," for example, the act of living is seen as an art form. You are given a body, certain limitations, certain assets and, within this framework, your life is a work of art, your own creation. To dull and tarnish it with essentially meaningless activity and unfulfillment is to copy but the ordinary. "We are trying to think in universal rather than fragmented terms. Communes are not freak historical phenomena; the communes are an affirmative response to a current hunger for community. They form, fold, reform, fade, die, get chased away, and try once again to re-form somewhere else. But they remain mutations in nature. And that's the way evolution works: millions of mutants come forth, struggle and die for every one fairly viable creature that carries on."

It is not our intention to paint an overly rosy and uncritical picture of communal life. Obviously, communes do attract others than those on a genuine personal quest. Some are permanent dropouts, not so much from work, but from life. Others are chasing a fantasy of free sex, lack of responsibility, an easy answer, or just trying to keep up on the latest fad—the fad defining them rather than they defining the fad. Elia Katz in *Armed Love* observed that commune-living children of rat-racing, square Scarsdale parents had as much greedy eagerness for popularity, male tyranny, ego assassination, sexual hypocrisy, social bullying, and escapism as their suburban parents.

### Chasing Fantasies

When work becomes unmeaningful, some chase more of the same—promotions, bigger houses, and better cars. Others chase fantasies. In discussing leisure, Ray Orrock points out, "Most of us do entertain a fantasy from time to time, putting our feet on the desk and gazing at the airline's calendar depicting a balmy tropical isle, thinking: 'Boy, if I could just get away to a place like that! No pressures—no hassles. Just lie in the sun, drink cool drinks and swim a little . . . all day long. What a life that would be!' " He then goes on to describe the experience of John Keffend, an editor for *Time Magazine*, who finally decided to give up his good job and nice home to move to Pago Pago, Samoa, where he lived inexpensively, swam daily, sipped and dined with friends until late at night, watched the sunset, enjoyed the children playing, wrote in his journal, and sunned daily on the beach. He spent two years carving out a life style in paradise, attaining what many men dream of, fulfilling a fantasy toward which many men strive all their lives and never realize. After two years, John Keffend came home, reporting, "Life in paradise is just too boring . . . and there was too much time there; you've got to figure out how to kill it." For those who chase the American dream, the dream of attaining a life of leisure in paradise, fantasizing the good life in a commune, or any other dream, the lesson to be learned may be that life is lived where you are at, right now, and "if you can't make it where you are, you can't make it anywhere—so stop running." It is often difficult to differentiate a change in life style based on fundamental value considerations and sound judgment from those choices which are merely running from, not toward, something. The clearest key is one's past. If one has a history of chasing fantasies, pursuing a dream and always finding it wanting, being continually dissatisfied, then change may be as much in the service of avoiding the present as seeking a better future.

Just as we can chase sexual fantasies, the masculinity or femininity fantasy, so too can we chase a work or life style fantasy. We have so many to choose from. Lewis Roderick, being somewhat cynical about the American dreamer, the American consumer of life styles, describes in *Human Behavior*: "Now! At last! The new fall lineup of the very latest plans and styles for satisfactory living together. The list includes a dazzling variety of sizes and shapes, options and accessories, never before made available to the general public—and the cost is surprisingly low. You pay your money and take your choice, and may you live happily ever after. Or at least until next Tuesday. . . . Open Marriage, Mini-Marriage, Multilateral Marriage, or Trial Marriage, or perhaps simply Honest Sex, Total Sex, or Desensitized Intimacy." Or these life styles may be creatively interchanged with various values: Roderick's "Getting Ahead, Fun Fervor, Creative Frenzy,

Mystic Withdrawal, Technique Infatuation," and so on. With so many life styles as possibilities, with so many fantasies to chase, one may be continually dissatisfied. The running away from life in search of a fantasy, continually being on a "Journey to the East," may often prevent rather than enhance a person's ability to make commitments about life style, work, play, and marriage. Alvin Toffler makes the point, "the commitment to one style of life over another is thus a super-decision. It is a decision of a higher order than the general run of everyday life decisions. It is a decision to narrow the range of alternatives that will concern us in the future . . . to be 'between styles' or 'between subcults' is a life crisis, and the people of the future spend more time in this condition searching for styles than do people of the past or present." The mere fact that more and more is being written about life styles indicates a growing interest in assessing one's total life, in not compartmentally isolating one's work from meaningfulness, in integrating rather than elevating one's success, money, and achievement needs in life. Such takes strength; such leads to strength.

### Integrating New Roles

Many new attempts at a more balanced expression of living have arisen out of the efforts of many strong women demanding their freedom to grow in relationship to the men in their lives. Just as many men become strong by learning to accept a working wife (although they may emotionally feel somewhat reluctant about it, as most men in our culture have been taught to feel), so too are many women accepting nonearning husbands. Many couples are becoming stronger in learning to respect the right of each other to personal growth through negotiating a suitable arrangement to satisfy the needs of each. This has resulted, for some, in a very traditional life arrangement with the wife staying home looking after the kids and the husband working, but it has resulted also in the reverse, or combinations of the two patterns. The emphasis is becoming less on traditional roles and more on the respect each has for the other as unique persons developing in ways each chooses for himself in the context of their relationship. Though not without many difficulties, the American couple, relative to those in many parts of the world, is adapting very quickly to new changes in traditional roles and expectations. In the process, women become stronger by treating men as persons rather than as providers; and men are becoming stronger by treating women as persons rather than as homemakers.

In the perspective of personhood and human needs, including needs for esteem and self-actualization, the question of work for men or women is of great relevance for fostering strength, because it is a question to be answered in the light of personal growth rather than as a concept rigidly tied to traditional roles and cultural expectations. A strong man is not afraid of working for a woman. A strong woman does not use a superior position to put down men.

### Living Your Learning

To become stronger necessitates struggle to overcome the negative aspects of your education (as Ivan Illich points out in *Deschooling Society*). We learn facts, not how to think. We learn techniques, not the implications of their application. The educational institutions that produce the strongest persons find ways of combining and helping to integrate more directly the student's learning with his living experience, and of fostering both inner and outer mastery.

Many "liberal arts" institutions, not only scientific and technical schools, "miss the boat" in fostering human development. Trying to provide a liberal education (to educate "the whole person"), they present information in the humanities and social sciences, with a sprinkling of physical and biological sciences and art—a large amount of unintegrated material. There are rarely classes on personal integration to help the student synthesize the information he has acquired. There are very few classes on personal values that help a student discover and implement systematically a set of values of his own. There are classes on the philosophy of others, but there are few classes on developing one's own philosophy. Schools expect the student to derive a set of values from his parents; the parents expect him to learn his values in church; and the student is bewildered because no one helps him to learn systematically to assess his personal experience in such a way as to find meaning (from which he might derive values) and a way to integrate his experience so as to make sense of competing and often conflicting ideologies. With the rigid separation of Church and State, many institutions studiously avoid any exploration of values (especially when they might be seen as ultimate ones); they may present the beliefs of others, but find it difficult to help a student explore his personal beliefs meaningfully.

### The Pursuit of Excellence

In the reaction against a mechanistic, dehumanized way of life, the pursuit of excellence has sometimes been lost in the shuffle. All of us would much prefer to be operated upon by a hostile, arrogant, well-trained and highly skilled surgeon than by a sloppy, technically incompetent one with a good bedside manner. Even for the psycho-therapist, whose self is a vital aspect of his professional armamentar-ium, being a kindly person is no substitute for a knowledge of the behavioral sciences.

A strong person is concerned with excellence. When work is an outer expression of inner harmony, quality and uniqueness are likely. The motivations of the strong toward excellence are different from those of the achievement-seeker, but some of the results can be the same. Though he values a breadth of activity, he rejects being a jack-of-all-trades and master of none. Just as a strong person tolerates, but does not seek, turmoil and distress, he can put up with necessary drudgery in the pursuit of a goal. He is dissatisfied with monotonous work, but knows that some aspects of work inevitably tend to be tedious. The old adage that creative research is "10 percent inspira-tion and 90 percent perspiration" holds true. The strong reduce frustration by the fulfillment of intrinsic potentialities in both work and play.

Although it may be true that many drop out in order to avoid work, it would be unreasonable to assume that, just because a person decides to earn his living doing crafts or working as a lifeguard, he is lazy. Youth is often accused of being lazy when, in fact, it is envied for enjoying its work. It used to be, for example, as pointed out by William Stephens, that "masterpieces were once as common as ordinary skilled craftsmen. For each craftsman had to produce a 'masterpiece' before he could be called a 'master' at his craft—his reward for fulfilling the work ethic of his era. . . . A would-be craftsman had to study under a master for seven years. Before the apprentice could be accepted into the guild, he had to fashion a masterpiece acceptable to his master." The point is that genuine and creative self-expression may require an incredible amount of work, training, and perspiration. The willingness of many persons to work—really work—at something they enjoy, without necessarily high pay, bespeaks a new generation of potentially very strong persons, willing to seek personal meaning and happiness above an unnecessary overkill in the seeking of security represented by money, social status, and success.

Jacqueline Bouhoutsos and Charles Ansell point out, "It is this psychological distance from work that measures the sense of job and the depth of meaning we derive from our occupations. The farther a person stands psychologically from his work, the less that work expresses him and the more meager are the rewards. Those fortunate enough to stand close to their work approach an inner integration. Without this closeness, we are in danger of becoming depersonalized, a state in which the sense of self, so essential to emotional well-being, undergoes serious fragmentation."

### Play

In our discussion of sex we have already commented upon the utility of and the strength required in "letting go"—and sex isn't the only way to play. The Protestant Ethic tends to make us feel guilty about frivolity. A product of this ethic tends to feel that he should be raking leaves, washing the car, or perusing a scientific journal when he sits down by his pool. A strong person is likely to retain an element of the child within him, able to express lightheartedness and playfulness, and able to be childlike without being childish.

Play, like sex, can be used for other goals. Competitiveness can be in the service of winning out—achieving power or fame rather than working in the service of excellence and self-fulfillment. We tend to work at play, to get our golf score into the low 80s with grim determination.

Play can be a gratifying way to enhance a sense of outer mastery, a way to seek challenge and thus gain confidence and become stronger. It can be a way to help us get in touch with our bodies. It can also enhance our relatedness to our teammates, opponents, or playmates.

For the strong, the distinction between work and play is often blurred. Their recreation not only refreshes, it re-creates their wholeness.

8

# PROBLEMS OF THE STRONG PERSON

Common to persons of habitual strength are some unique and essentially intrinsic problems. These major problems arise precisely out of strength, of being seen by others as being "strong," of allowing oneself to be perceived as a "strong person," and out of one's commitment to being humane. Although it may seem surprising, it is not uncommon to find in the life of a person who typically behaves in fashions that can be defined as strong such recurrent feelings as loneliness, frustration, disappointment, sadness, resentment, and a sense of being overburdened and overextended. Many pitfalls lie in the path of the typically strong. If they are not avoided or surmounted, the strong become less strong, they are weakened.

### Being an Idol

If a person is frequently strong, others seek to draw on his strength, seek his counsel and advice, draw on his experience to aid themselves in their own personal growth, and solicit his help in times of need. The more often he exhibits strength, the less others see his personal problems, his anxieties, and his own troubles. They tend to expect always to receive support from him. Signs of weakness will often be ignored or unnoticed because they are incongruous with the image of a "strong person." Or, in genuine moments of need, a generally strong person may turn to one that he has often helped. Not infrequently, this other person will become frightened, angry, and turn away. Having seen mostly strength, having drawn on that strength, any sign of weakness or humanness may be confusing or frightening. He may even report to friends later how disillusioning it was to find that his so-called "strong person" was not everything he was cracked up to be, that he indeed had feet of clay.

## Fear of Strong Persons

Many people who are not very self-contained, who have many problems, who are relatively outer-directed, do not often consider or dare to take a stronger person into relationship with themselves. It may not occur to them that they could do so. The need of a stronger person to be helped or cared for may, for many people, be frightening. They may fear engulfment by the stronger, or they may see their source of stability and strength in the world suddenly crumbling. Often needing someone to stand between them and the harshness of the world, needing the stronger person almost as a parent or protector, they may avoid perceiving a strong person as being needful or vulnerable. To do so would be to deprive themselves of a supporting pillar in life. Furthermore, they may fear that the stronger person would not value what they have to offer. So, during those times when a strong person needs to be cared for, comforted, and rewarded, others are not apt to notice or, if noticing, may not feel as though they can be of help.

## The Victim of High Expectations

A person used to acting out of strength may come to expect too much of himself. Always being seen as strong by others, he may come to expect of himself that he does not need others. Typically giving, continually ministering to others, being constantly looked to by others as a source of strength, he may come to see himself as stronger and more self-contained than he is in reality. Perceiving himself thus, it may become incongruous for him to ask for help or to reveal his times of need. During times of "weakness" or turmoil, he will often have unmet needs, unmet in part because he does not consider the possibility that those he has frequently aided can be of help to him. It is not uncommon for him to feel isolated, lonely, drained of strength, and, during these times to come to resent those who always take and himself for always giving. His resentment may be enhanced because he considers himself to be deserving. Yet he may not give others a chance.

Furthermore, a person of seemingly continual strength may expect of others what he himself is capable of giving: concern, commitment, warmth, ability, and so on. He is not a hypocrite in that he himself would be willing to give what he expects, but he may be unrealistic in his expectations. Strength is relatively rare. He may also alienate others and drive them away through his disappointment in their poor performance relative to his expectations, thus increasing his relative isolation in times of need.

### *Overcommitment*

A person of considerable strength often finds himself in the position of making too many commitments. He undertakes a variety of tasks. He may be frequently called upon because of his skills and effectiveness, not only because of his concern and compassion. He may find it hard to say "no," not out of a propensity toward compliance, but out of generosity, helpfulness, and readiness to undertake challenge. Each activity or relationship may be genuinely rewarding, interesting, or enjoyable, but the combination can be overwhelming. Fatigue and exhaustion set in. A sense of being overburdened and resentful may ensue. His enthusiasm about the present may lead to involvements that mortgage the future, leading to diminished energy reserves, diminished personal strength. The difficult skill of being able to say no must be mastered in order continually to function as a strong person.

A colleague called in sick one day, more dispirited than he had been in years, burdened down by a series of emergencies at work and crises at home. He needed to have the day just alone, to gather his strength and minister to himself. He told the secretary, "I feel really old today. I am just going to sit in my rocker all day." Two hours did not go by before he got a panic call from a client who desperately needed him. For the first time in their relationship, he told her that he did not have any energy, anything left to give that day, that he was utterly exhausted, and could she possibly see him the next day. She said "O.K." but an hour later she called back, more insistent than ever that she needed help "right now." Having taken some responsibility for this person and having convinced himself that her plight was real, he finally drove the forty miles necessary to see her, ministered to her needs while almost crying to himself, wondering how his own needs would be met.

### The Martyr's Trap

It is common for a strong person to establish a self-image as a giving person, as a loving person who always thinks of others without thought of personal gain. In doing so, however, he may set himself up for failure, for he may be requiring himself to be what he is not: a faultless, altruistic person. It will be difficult for him to accept the giving of others, for he must be the giver. He will have difficulty in sharing his sadness and anger and other unwanted feelings, for this would be inconsistent with his image of himself as an altruistic person. Thus, he may deny others the opportunity of giving to him, of doing in their lives the very thing he demands of himself: helping and giving. Because he may then find it inconsistent to express many parts of himself, more and more he will have less and less to give, for his energies will be increasingly bound up with loose ends, unexpressed and unshared parts of himself. The danger at these moments is that the person of strength will continue to hide his feelings and feel sorry for himself and in the process become less strong. If he cannot share these feelings with others in a direct way, then he may fall prey to the martyr's trap and again be led away from the path of strength.

### Fear of Being Overwhelmed

A further trap exists for those who are perceived by others as being strong in that they may often seem overwhelming and frightening to others. Others may find it difficult to assert themselves in relationship to such a person. His affection may appear to demand too much in return. They may feel engulfed by his personal power. They may fear loss of their own identity in juxtaposition to the strength of his. Others may distance themselves from a strong person for self-protection, leading to his isolation. The strong may heighten their feelings of inadequacy or inferiority. When the otherwise strong lose sight of this fact, they may often inadvertently find themselves alone and feeling lonely.

### A Victim of Projection

It is easy for others to misperceive the motives and feelings underlying the behavior of a strong person, with which they may be unfamiliar relative to their own experience. His directness may seem critical. His giving may be seen as phony, manipulative, or demanding. It is hard to believe in generosity and empathy, especially if you lack these traits yourself. You ask, "What's in it for him?"

### Fear of Exposure

Others may also fear being "seen through," by having their weaknesses revealed in the presence of a stronger person. The more strong a person is, the more perceptive he tends to be, but he is not a mind-reader. More importantly, others may not appreciate his capacity for acceptance or his ability to withhold judgment. A person truly strong is not critical, but is likely to have others' self-criticalness projected upon him. Those perfectionists and high achievers who seem strong and yet critically give others a hard time, are really among the "pseudo-strong."

Thus, for those who are frequently strong and tend subsequently to be perceived as and related to as "strong persons," a special set of problems arises in which it may be difficult for them consistently to get their own needs met. Loneliness and needfulness are common but infrequently recognized in the strong. Those of strength are often, like every person, in need of help, affection, and caring.

# 9

# HELPING A
# STRONG PERSON

We all relate to the strengths within ourselves and others. In developing our own strength, we must be able both to seek help from others and to know how to help ourselves. In encountering the strong, we must find ways to meet their often hidden needs, to enhance their satisfaction and to further their growth, and in the process become stronger ourselves.

## HELPING YOURSELF TO BE STRONGER

### Seek Others of Strength

If you characteristically behave in strong ways, there will be times when you need to turn to someone respected, someone who is reliably secure enough to be in a position to help. There are some areas of experience, some of the things about yourself, that can be best understood and empathized with by another strong person, someone who is more apt to know the kinds of struggles that are unique to stronger people, someone who can be relied upon not to be threatened by self-disclosures, anger, or resentment. In relationship to another person of strength, you are apt to get consistent and reliable feedback about yourself. There is a sense of security in knowing that there is someone else who can be of help consistently, without fostering dependency.

In some ways, none of us outgrow the need for the parent who was always able to protect us, to stand between us and the outside world. In our times of deepest trouble and internal turmoil, we all tend to turn to someone who functions as or represents that parent, someone who has control of things when we do not, someone stronger than we are. Strong people need each other for those special times when they themselves need the protection and strength they have often given others. None of us is so strong that we do not sometimes feel inadequate, that we are not sometimes overwhelmed by events beyond our control.

### Look to Those Frequently Less Strong

It helps to realize that there are times when others who are usually less strong will in fact be stronger than yourself. Strength is a relative concept, changing from moment to moment. Although a person typically may be less strong than yourself, there will be times when he is in a stronger relative position. Strength, after all, is an abstraction, not representing a "thing" or a fixed point on a continuum, but rather a way of behaving or relating in a particular situation or to a particular person. Between two people at any given moment in time, the less needful one, the one more able to give of himself, the one whose resources at that particular time permit courage, the one less in conflict, is the stronger. This interpersonal system is fluid and may readily shift. Strength is required to acknowledge that you are now in a temporarily less strong position. Such lack of strength is not "bad," merely human. If you habitually condemn yourself for always being in the "weaker" position, you deny your humanity and thus are not truly strong.

### Acknowledge "Weakness"

You become stronger by acknowledging weakness. The competitiveness of our culture, the emphasis on winning, on who is first, or on who is better than another, tends to separate people, tends to categorize those who are less strong, who are "weaker," as somehow being unworthy. Part of becoming stronger is in establishing communality with humanity, sharing collective involvement in life and transcending artificial distinctions that tend to separate rather than integrate.

The individual who displays his "strength" as a sign of superiority certainly is not being strong.

An encounter group leader, having given much of himself during a "sensitivity weekend," found himself overwhelmed by feelings of loneliness, stimulated by a group exercise. Having discerned his need for closeness, two people moved to him and held him. They were, in fact, two young freshman girls he had somewhat condescendingly labeled as being the most frail and weak persons in the group—so different from himself. "You know," he said afterward, "that experience was awfully good for me. It brought me back down to earth. It may really be that most people are confused, mixed up, neurotic, or weak. But it doesn't really matter. I need those people."

### Avoid Encouraging a "Strong Image"

Likewise, if you are stereotyped as "strong" and if your "real self" is sad, troubled, worried, or even joyful or affectionate, it helps to know that you are presenting a gift of yourself if you share this (for the moment) "real self" with those who are close. This sharing is meaningful and often more appreciated than the perceived "strength" that is projected most of the time. The seemingly self-sufficient, being perceived as unneedy, often put others off, awakening in them feelings of inadequacy in the face of their own human needfulness. The hero with the fatal flaw, the saint who falls at times, are characters in life and literature the more beloved for their weaknesses (humanness). The old saying is that "one can never love a saint." It is equally true that it is very difficult to love a person who always seems strong, never needing.

For the longest time, I (JAK) couldn't discover why I felt nothing toward an obviously attractive, bright, and verbal intern, the top of her class. Then, one day during a long conversation, she told me with some feeling how she had difficulty coping with the fact that she had greater needs for expressing affection than did her husband. As I felt a flood of warmth for her, it dawned on me that this was her first disclosure to me that revealed her humanness, that showed she didn't have "everything together." I also found myself being more comfortable because I could more easily share some of my struggles, knowing that she could, indeed, empathize.

### Share Your Ideas and Activities

You have more than your feelings to share. People have their interests, philosophies, beliefs, ideals and perceptions of reality. Besides feelings and thoughts, there are actions and activities. A relatively strong person may at times find it hard to be understood. His view may be highly personal or socially unconventional. There is excitement in intellectual exchange and intuitive mutual understanding as well as in transactions on a more emotional level. Without being arrogant or dogmatic, a strong person lets others in on how he sees the world and may often serve as an educator in opening up new perspectives to those of more limited vision. You enrich yourself and allow others more awareness of yourself through bringing them into contact with your "doing" self, whether it is in the area of gliding, organic gardening, handball, weaving, or analyzing the stock market.

### Allow Others to Give to You

There is something unsettling and anxiety-provoking in always receiving from another. It is common to come to resent and dislike those who always give and never allow repayment. It makes a person feel like a child to be constantly beholden to another for help or favors without being provided a way to be useful in return. No one likes to be continually in debt. Strength is required to ask advice on personal problems, to ask how to handle troubling relationships, to ask how you are coming across. If you need a favor, can you allow someone to be inconvenienced? A strong person knows how to receive as well as to give. Both giver and recipient are enhanced by mutuality.

Too, your own welfare is bound up with that of mankind. The growth of another person is beneficial to you, for it helps mankind take a small step forward to greater collective strength and harmony. Other people come to see themselves as being stronger as they relate to strength. In this sense, you contribute to the growth of another by allowing the other to be of help.

### Monitor Your Time Priorities

A strong person, often the center of a busy life, bound up with developing external as well as internal skills, wanting to be of help to others, simply finding himself overcommitted, may discover that his family is the first cut on the priority list because of less enjoyable but more "important" demands. This leads to the neglecting of important sources of interpersonal strength found in intimacy. In recognizing intimacy needs as important and in giving them priority accordingly, commitment to their fulfillment ensues. Commitment is represented by the time cleared to be close with others, to share with spouse, children, and friends. If married, for example, it is possible consciously to plan to spend a half-hour or so daily just in personal sharing of yourself with your spouse. A block of time each week might well be set aside with each child alone, just listening and sharing affections and frustrations in relationship to him. Friends, too, need "quality time" together.

## HELPING A TYPICALLY STRONG OTHER

### Infer His Needfulness

Many sons and daughters, even as adults, look at their parents and ask themselves, "What can I possibly give to them?" Many people work for a relatively strong, competent person who seems so skilled and knowledgeable that it strains the imagination to discern ways to enrich his or her life or be in any way helpful. Many people have a strong, nurturing mother, always a source of comfort and affection. She seems to have an unending supply of caring and energy for those she loves. Who can give anything to such a person except gratitude and love? Many of us relate to a person who is well-known or is a family hero. Even if we have considerable contact with such a person, he or she may seem unreachable, to be viewed from a distance and deferred to, but certainly not seen as needing help. As we have pointed out, success is not necessarily proof of strength, but, assuming such successful persons are indeed strong in other ways too, how can we be of help to them? One device is to assume that the apparently strong person has needs much the same as your own. When times of tiredness, unusual aloofness, remoteness, or irritability are noted, they can be mentioned. A strong person needs to know that you can be of help.

It is a trap, however, to feel you must give concretely and specifically to a stronger person in order to *deserve* his or her affection or to feel that you are obligated to repay. A strong person finds gratification in his helpfulness for its own sake and in the enhancement of self-esteem that results from living up to his ideals of how to treat others. Mutuality of helpfulness does not mean "tit for tat," getting and giving, being helped and helping back directly. Just as the child of generous parents can only repay by being a good parent himself, the recipient of the largesse of a stronger person can repay humanity, can give to those now in need, as he has once received.

Thus, the strong person's contribution to mankind can be multiplied indirectly through the actions of those he has benefited.

## Be Forward with Your Honesty

All grow strong in their honesty. It is strength that allows you to share your frustrations about a strong person with him. If you feel hurt by never being allowed to be of service to the strong person, tell him. In doing so, you will be developing your own strength, presenting your real self, and sharing real feelings (even of frustration or inadequacy). As such, you are really giving a strong person the gift of yourself. At a particular level, self-disclosure begets similar disclosures at that level. Most people will respond at the same level of disclosure presented to them. Thus, if one is asked, "Isn't it a lovely day outside?" he is apt to reply, "Yes, the temperature is perfect." "How is your sick mother?" is apt to elicit, "Feeling a little better, thank you." If he is told, "I enjoy being around you," he will probably respond with comments about feelings he has about you. In the long run, you tend to get what you give, whether the person is stronger or not.

## Acknowledge Your Fears of the Stronger Person

Fear of engulfment by the stronger person can keep us from reaching out to him. It is possible to reduce these risks, however, by focusing on the fact that a stronger person, too, has human needs. Focusing on his possible needs and away from your own anxiety allows greater latitude to act. Another tactic is to tell yourself that it is all right to have these feelings as long as they do not alter appropriate behavior. If such feelings are consistently part of a relationship to someone stronger, then revelation and mutual working through can help overcome the anxieties. A person acting out of strength will not attack when you reveal to him what appears to be a weakness, especially when there is an evident effort to overcome that "weakness." Such a revelation will serve to aid in developing yourself as a stronger person by being real and thus intrinsically more worthwhile and important to the already strong person. Such revelation also helps a strong person to be more sensitive to the anxieties he elicits in others. There is always more strength in accepting a weakness or unwanted feeling and acknowledging it in relationship to another than in denying it. Anyone can remain hidden; it takes strength to reveal oneself.

# 10

# FOSTERING STRENGTH IN CHILDREN

The best teacher is generally the best model of what he teaches. Parents teach their child most effectively by modeling the behaviors that reflect their values, their standards, and their philosophies of life. The parent who is a good example of that which he values (although he may rarely speak explicitly of his values) will have far more influence on his children than the parent who moralizes and lectures his child, attempting to mold and shape him, yet providing an inconsistent or poor model of those values. The attempt to create strong children, similarly, is best made by being a model of strength rather than trying to teach strength to the child. To foster strength in a child, then, may require self-modification of parental behavior as well as efforts to influence the behavior of the child and to provide him with suitable challenges.

### Discovering versus Molding Strength

A child's strength must come from within himself; it cannot be given him from without. This knowledge is highly significant; it implies that you must have trust in your child's resources, that you must relate to the strengths within the child. It is antithetical to this orientation and easy to assume that you "own" your children, or "possess" them, or are responsible for "molding" or "indoctrinating" them with what is right and proper. Rules, doctrines, values, and attitudes that tend to be imposed from without (beaten into the child either physically or psychologically) will not foster strength in the child, for they deprive him of the opportunity to rely on his own resources, his own developing strengths, and his own experience from which he will eventually be able to derive and integrate his own values, attitudes, and preferences in life. Rather than imposing specific values and standards, parents need to imply that it is important to *have* values and to live up to them. If the child is not allowed to develop his own resources consistently, he will not have acquired the skill and emotional autonomy to become an independent, self-reliant person as an adult. It is necessary for developing strength in a child to relate to and trust in the strength that the child possesses. As Abraham Maslow points out, "It seems quite clear that all organisms are more self-regulating and autonomous than we thought 25 years ago. The organism deserves a good deal of trust."

Just as there is no one pattern of psychological strength and no given way to be strong, there is no single pattern leading to the development of strength during childhood. Sometimes the most difficult childhoods produce the strongest and most remarkable people. It sometimes appears as if adversity "makes or breaks." Challenges too great for the adaptive capacity and maturational level of the child are destructive, while lack of challenge stultifies development. A professional colleague had the great compliment of having one of his students say, "My wife is pregnant with our first child. Since I admire and respect you so greatly, I would like to know how your parents reared you, so that our kid will turn out to be the kind of person you are." In reporting this incident, our colleague said, "I was really moved, but I just didn't know what to say. I rarely ever reveal this, but I was a 'battered child.' My father broke my leg twice. My mother is a drunk who still shows little interest in me and my children. Should I have told him to beat his child? I really don't know how I managed to turn out okay. I guess I had to struggle through life and thus gained confidence. I've always been sensitive to suffering. Then, too, I was smart and had a lot of good people outside the home that helped me along the way."

### Fostering Inner Strength: Trust and Security

Earlier, we characterized the strong person as having inner, interpersonal, and outer masteries. Helping a child develop a sense of inner mastery in general is a vague and abstract notion. As we look at some of the characteristics of the strong person that bespeak inner mastery, what a parent might do to create this mastery becomes somewhat more apparent.

Personal security and basic trust of others are prerequisites of psychological strength. As parents, we create personal security and trust in our children by both consciously and intuitively meeting their needs. Infants have needs for food, warmth, touch, affection, and the many other basic physiological and psychological needs. These needs are always important to the child but never as crucial as in his first months of life when he is totally dependent on his parents for sensing and meeting these needs. Only if these needs are accurately perceived and consistently and reliably attended to will he come to have trust in his environment, to feel secure that these needs will continue to be met, and to develop the rudiments of faith in others that will enable him later to relate more successfully to others. Well-meaning parents can, however, misinterpret an infant's distress signals. For example, one of the hypothesized causes of obesity in later life is some parents' tendency to automatically feed a baby whenever he cries—the child comes to associate feeding with the amelioration of any subjective discomfort. (An obese client lamented "in our house, food was love.") Erik Erikson describes this earliest period in a child's life as crucial in laying the foundation for a life of either basic trust or basic mistrust. Only when the child perceives the environment as consistently, predictably, and accurately meeting his needs can he learn to delay gratification, secure that it will be forthcoming.

Especially during the early months of a child's life, there is the temptation to say as parents: "Well, what about my needs? I want my kid to respect my need to sleep, to be undisturbed by crying. He can eat when I eat. He might as well start now learning that we have dinner at 6:00 and breakfast at 7:00." Although it is important for a child to eventually learn to respect the needs of others, he must learn to do this at an age when it is possible for him to be both empathetic and responsive to such needs.

Even more malignant than rigidity is the parent's confusion of his or her needs with those of the child—for example, the mother's feeding the child when she is hungry rather than when the baby appears to want to eat. Such a process, when compounded by later similar projections, may be a factor in the confusion of ego boundaries and difficulty in handling inner drive states characteristic of schizophrenic illnesses. If the child is not able to trust his human environment, the groundwork will be laid for suspiciousness, greed, insatiability, dependency, oversensitivity, apathy, or withdrawal as neurotic ego traits resulting from failure and attempts at repair or defense in regard to earliest developmental tasks. Too, as Maslow has pointed out, if a person's basic physiological needs and his needs for safety and security are not met, then he may be chronically stuck at that need level. Not being secure, for example, he will not be free to move up to meet his other needs for love and belongingness and from there to move on to even higher needs. Thus, not meeting an infant's basic needs may result in varying degrees of insecurity that will hamper and distort later stages of psychosexual growth and impair development of higher needs. Developmental failures, which can result from a variety of deprivations or overindulgences, can lead to "fixation" at a particular state of development, hampering further growth and leaving the individual with residuals of infantile conflicts and behavior throughout life. In the presence of severe life stress, there is always a tendency to regress to previous points of fixation.

## *Fostering Self-Awareness and Self-Acceptance*

Inner mastery includes being self-aware, self-accepting, having a personal sense of worth and being more inner- than outer-directed. Helping a child to develop these attributes is a task that begins when a child is an infant and continues through the many developmental crises and stages that he must undergo before leaving home. A child becomes self-aware and self-accepting when a parent takes time to "tune in" on his feelings, listens to them, names them and accepts them without judging, evaluating, putting down, or lecturing about or demanding logic of these feelings. For example, a child left behind by an older sibling might be asked: "Do you feel unwanted?" A child does not come into the world with a vocabulary for distinguishing among his feelings—they are at the beginning an undifferentiated mass of emotions to him. Some of his feelings may frighten or overwhelm him. The parent, by consistently listening to, helping name, and nonjudgmentally accepting and understanding a child's feelings, does many things for him at the same time:

> He helps the child develop a vocabulary so he can differentiate among his inner feelings. This process aids transition from perceptual to conceptual thinking, as already stated, which moves him toward control and mastery.

He helps the child listen to and understand what he is feeling.

He helps the child learn that his feelings are important. The strong parent values his own feelings, but he came to this stage because others have listened to and understood and been interested in those feelings. So, too, must he do for his children.

If the parent is accepting of a child's feelings and does not get defensive and angry, the child learns that it is all right for him to have feelings—he is enabled to accept his own feelings.

If the parent does not judge the child's feelings or try to lecture to the child or point out how illogical his feelings are, the child then will not come to expect his feelings to be logical (an important attribute of the strong person) and he will not feel guilty for having feelings; they will be acceptable to him because they are acceptable to others. His behaviors may cause others problems, for which he will have to take eventual responsibility, but his feelings are just feelings, not things to be felt guilty about, criticized for, or put down.

All a child knows of the world is his own experience. When others, like his parents, find his experience worthy of attention and interest, the child comes to feel that he and his own experience are indeed worthwhile.

Putting down a child's feelings is all too easy. It almost comes naturally: "How can you be ungrateful to your grandmother after all she has done for you?" "What do you mean—you feel bored? This is the best parade the town has had in years." "You think I've been unfair to you? What a stupid thing to feel—I'm always fair with all my kids." "Big boys don't cry." "Don't worry about it—everything will be all right." "Don't be mad at your mother. Children should respect their parents." "Wipe that look off your face!" All these are messages saying that the child's feelings are wrong or illegitimate or not valid. The child needs to have his feelings (although not necessarily his behavior) understood and accepted. (Accepting the child's feelings is not synonymous with permissiveness. Parents often lecture, moralize, demand logic of, become angry at, or avoid confronting the child's feelings. Unfortunately, this is at the expense of the child's needs to be heard, understood, and accepted; consequently he will not come to accept his own feelings, will not be secure in sharing himself with others later in life, and will not have the skills for mastering his own inner life. The parent who tends to send the above messages may also inadvertently be modeling a lack of knowledge of and acceptance of his own feelings, which causes him to find it difficult to understand and accept the feelings of others (including his children). One cannot teach well what one does not live.

## Fostering Interpersonal Strength

There comes a time when a child is capable of responding to the needs and feelings of his parents. As he grows older, he may at some point understand a tired father's need to have fewer cowboys and Indians around the fort. A significant shift for an infant occurs when he moves from a state of total dependency in which all his needs are met to a time when he must also respond to the needs and expectations of others. How the parents handle this transition has significant impact on the child.

## The Child of Power-Oriented Parents

Power-oriented parents, when they want their children to respond to their needs, resort to their power and authority—they make a decision about what the child is going to do, and then tell him or cause him to do it. "Shut the door." "Stop that racket!" "Go to your room and don't come out until I tell you." "Don't ask me for a ride to school—ride your bike." Parents have much power and authority. Yet a child, too, must develop his own sense of self and his own sense of power and initiative. Even a young child can sense that through the use of power the parent is satisfying his own needs at the expense of his own, and that seems unfair. The parent's use of power over a child also teaches him that his own needs are not very important. Children often rebel against authority, using such tactics as defiance, opposition, or passive aggression. Defiance can lead to rebelliousness that later causes trouble with authorities. The misuse of parental authority is in fact a problem of major proportions. For authoritarian parents, childhood defiance can lead to frustration, with consequent rage, abuse, and rejection. Power is used by parents who know of no other way of getting their wishes met. The child, as a result, does not learn to respect or want to fulfill the needs of others. He is significantly blocked from growing stronger because one of the major characteristics of strength is that of being able to respond to the needs of others—being able to give. Interestingly, the power-oriented parent is often the first to complain about a son or daughter's lack of respect and inconsiderateness when it seems that they would be proud to have children so much like themselves—adept in the use of power. Children who learn to put their needs before those of others use their increasing stores of power against their parents and others.

Similarly handicapped is the child who responds to parental

authority with submission, compliance, and passivity. This child learns to put down his own needs in deference to others. He may also be bashful, perfectionistic, and outer-directed, performing for others in order to feel worthwhile rather than being inner-directed and choosing how to behave in light of both his own needs and the needs of others. This type is, in some respects, the model of the "all-American" boy or girl, who does everything well, is eager to please others, yet lacks a sense of inner direction, autonomy, and self-confidence stemming from an inner sense of what he wants and is capable of and an awareness of the needs of others.

### The Child of the Permissive Parent

The permissive parent follows the other model so commonly used with children. The permissive parent that tends to sacrifice his own needs rather than those of his children. He or she is a martyr of sorts, sacrificing everything for the child, always giving, self-sacrificing, selfless, "altruistic," all-loving, in some ways a model of what many consider to be virtuous and good, the *magna mater* ("big momma"). Yet the results in the children may not be as planned. The child who always gets his way does not know how to respect the feelings of others. Because the parent does not respect his own needs and feelings enough to assert them in relationship to his children, the children certainly do not learn to respect them on their own. The child-centered home may produce the free-loader, the uncooperative and unmanageable bully, the manipulator, the sociopath who transgresses against others without feelings of guilt or remorse, never having learned the extent or nature of his impact on others. Lack of control and of conscience is one outcome of permissiveness. Excessive guilt can be another. The child never limited by the self-sacrificing parents can feel unworthy and self-punitive. The permissive parent may feel that there is greater virtue in his giving in than in the authoritarian's use of coercion and power.

Some parents attempt to combine the two methods, shifting first from one to another, leading to even greater confusion and conflict than the consistent use by both parents of either an authoritarian or a permissive approach. When one parent is authoritarian, one permissive, the "lenient" parent often becomes the "good guy," setting the stage for parental conflict and confusion in the child's determination of "right" behavior.

## A Democratic Model

A parent can use a democratic model, in which the feelings of both the child and parent are accepted and the behaviors which cause each other problems are negotiated so as to best meet the needs of both. In this regard, the parents need to take the initiative and be the models. They see that both their own needs and those of their children are important; both parents and children in this case can express their needs, acknowledge the needs of others, and thus be free to negotiate solutions acceptable and beneficial to everyone.

By taking the attitude that both his own feelings and the feelings of the child are important and need to be understood and that some kind of negotiation can take place in which a solution will be sought that would make them both happy, the parent accomplishes several things at once. He teaches the child that his needs are important, helping the child thus to develop a sense of worth and independence. He also teaches the child to recognize and respect the feelings of others, thus making him capable of modifying his own behavior for the good of someone else. This is different from compliance; it is problem-solving. The democratic model contains key ingredients for the development of strength in a child.

The task of listening to and respecting a child's feelings and teaching him to be aware of the needs and feelings of others is, of course, a difficult one for parents who were born and reared in homes with various mixtures of permissiveness and authoritarianism. Thomas Gordon in *Parent Effectiveness Training* treats intricacies of this difficult task in detail. *The Intimate Enemy* by George Bach gives a slightly different, but also useful, slant on dealing with one's own needs in relationship to those of others in his descriptions of nondestructive "fight training."

## Identity Formation

Those with inner strength have a firm sense of identity—they know who they are, where they are at, and what they believe, as well as having a sense of autonomy and independence. As mentioned earlier, a young child tends to shape much of his sense of identity as a man or a woman in relationship to his or her parent of the same sex. (This is relevant to parent-surrogates as well as to biological parents.) In some respects, as pointed out, identity formation is somewhat easier for a girl. Nurtured by a mother who met her early primary needs, the girl can identify with and receive affection from her mother through all of her childhood. The boy child, too, typically meets his early primary needs through his mother, yet must achieve his sense of sexual identity from his father. He must make a transition at some point that his sister does not have to make. This transition may often become rocky and represent a developmental crisis. The boy who has not resolved his "Oedipal" rivalry with the father over the mother's affections (generally because of his mother's rejection or seductiveness or because of father's hostility or passivity) finds it difficult to identify with his father. The boy whose father is competitive with him has a hard time resolving any intrinsic competitiveness with the father.

A further aspect of the child's identity formation comes from his or her relationship with the parent of the opposite sex. If the child feels comfortable and warm in relationship to that parent, he or she will be significantly influenced in his development as a heterosexual person. An opposite-sex parent who is respectful of and sensitive to both his own and the child's needs will pave the way for the child's being comfortable when giving and receiving affection from a significant person of the opposite sex. Without this kind of relationship, the child may have a difficult time relating to persons of the opposite sex as a young adult or adolescent.

Obviously, but often not admittedly, children are not an unmitigated blessing; they are often a big bother, not always the little bundles of joy they are "supposed" to be. Babysitters are needed. Adult activities are curtailed. Kids are expensive. They cause worry. They raise new doubts about parents' adequacy in their new roles. They reactivate parents' unresolved conflicts from their own childhoods. Parents can resent children's competitiveness for the time and attention of the spouse. (Such rivalries, of course, often have deeper sexual and pregenital implications.) Unless all these feelings are discussed and resolved within the marriage itself, they may become directed to destructive attitudes and behaviors that prevent healthy identity formation in children. If parents are not aware of the range of their feelings engendered by having children in their lives, harbored resentments and hostilities, some of which may be directed toward the children, frequently make it more difficult for the child successfully to model himself after the parent. Parents who themselves did not have good parental models are particularly handicapped. Those deprived as children may find it hard to give to children. If a child feels that he is not getting enough of his mother's time, he needs to be listened to. If a father feels he is not getting enough of his wife's time, he needs to be listened to. Need conflicts between parents and children may result in competition and resentment. If parents are not sensitive to the very natural negative feelings they may have toward their children and the feelings that their children may naturally have in return, difficulty may arise. If the needs of all parties are respected, understood, and negotiated, the process of the child's identifying with his or her same-sex parent and achieving a positive identification is smoothed.

Previously, we have touched upon the complexity and difficulty of issues of masculinity and femininity, particularly the limitations of rigid traditional definitions. Obviously the same-sex parent serves as a model of sex-specific behaviors for identification by the child. New "unisex" patterns, working mothers, fathers who help around the home provide potentiality both for liberation and for confusion. The parents' security and sense of wholeness within themselves and their lack of competitiveness with each other will help. To treat the little girl globally as a fragile, emotional doll in pink ribbons, which limits her drive for competence and instrumental skills is just as thwarting as wishing she were a boy and encouraging only her activities in team sports, which devalues and does violence to her own feminine strivings. Parents more helpfully can be interested in the traits or qualities exhibited by the little boy or girl as his or her own—competence, achievement, curiosity about machines, interest in sports, as well as expression of feelings or artistic interests. The consistent validation of personhood, the enhancement of growth from within, will help produce an integrated human being, a strong person whose most basic traits provide commonality with humankind and who, as such, is more competent in relating to others as the man or woman he or she is.

### Being Intimate

In relationship to giving and receiving affection, strong persons have been characterized as being capable of engaging in intimate behavior—of sharing themselves. A parent can do three things that will help the child enhance his potential for intimacy. As already mentioned, he can listen nonjudgmentally to his child's expressed feelings, good or bad, hostile or caring. By tuning in and taking interest in these feelings, he encourages the child to trust that he can share all of himself without worrying about being judged, criticized, evaluated, or put down, a trust that is necessary to help him develop inner mastery and the potential for intimacy. The parent can also share with the child his own feelings, positive and negative, allowing the child to respond to his needs when appropriate, feeling his affection and caring when it is present. And, again, the parent in his model of intimacy with other members of the family and friends will provide an atmosphere where the child can observe intimacy, feel its effects, and learn by watching and practicing intimate behavior in relationship to his parents, siblings, and friends. Children identify not only with parents as individuals but often also with the quality of the relationship between them. How many children see their parents hug? How many see how parents are having and resolving conflicts?

### Fostering Outer Mastery

As soon as the infant can come to exert influence on his environment, he begins to achieve outer mastery. The use of language to help him more easily make his needs known and to get from others what he wants, the use of the toilet and of a toothbrush, the ability to open doors, turn on lights, tie shoes, and use the telephone are all tasks in which the young child can come to feel a sense of mastery.

When the child comes to direct more of his attention outside the family to others in the world—teachers, schoolmates, and others of his own age—he continues to meet new challenges, find new tasks to complete and new arenas in which he might fail. The early school years are often exciting times for children, filled with exploration, adventure, challenges, and new tasks. Experience here does much to help a child to feel either a sense of mastery or of failure. A small girl returning home from kindergarten sobbed, "I got an 'F' in school today, I know I did. I saw the teacher mark it down." At the teacher-parent conference the following week, the mother inquired about the "F"—it was there, all right, on the line marked, "Sex: M—— F——" This simple example shows that even a five-year-old recognizes the pressure to "do well." Are we pushing our children too far too fast, developing a whole generation of tense youngsters pressured to succeed in an increasingly competitive society?

Parents are in the difficult position of helping their children cope with a complex existence filled with competition and accelerating change. For a child to feel confident and masterful, he needs to successfully complete tasks that are set before him. He needs to be challenged, but not overwhelmed. Trying to make a six-year-old read a book designed for eight-year-olds when he is not ready, for example, may cause him to perceive himself as a failure. On the other hand, if the child is never challenged by his toys, his household tasks, his lessons, or in other areas of his life, then he never learns to cope with frustration or anxiety. Frustration, anxiety, and difficult tasks need to be introduced gradually into a child's life to provide him with challenge, but not at so great a pace as to overwhelm and create in him a sense of failure. If a child learns more slowly than others, he needs to be allowed to learn at his own pace. Pressing him to go faster is the way to stifle him and create feelings of failure.

As pointed out, strength in part is the sum of one's masteries minus the sum of one's failures. If a child never fails, however, he has not discovered his limitations, a necessity for self-knowledge. A child's failure, followed by a parent's understanding and acceptance of the failure, is a requisite for his later being able to accept failure as a natural and inevitable part of life. The child who is continually criticized, prodded, put down for doing poorly comes to fear failure; his chances for developing personal strength are undermined. The ability to accept failure is an important aspect of strength. Such acceptance is not the same as defeatism and actually fosters mastery.

## The Evaluation Trap

It is easy to evaluate a child unwittingly. Certain kinds of praise, for example, can be a subtle form of evaluation which can become internalized commands: "You're a good girl." "You're a nice young man." "You're a great runner—you'll be a champion some day." "You're so sweet and ladylike." The distinction is subtle, but there is a difference between praise and appreciation. In reality, you cannot know what is inside another person, what precisely he thinks or feels. What you do know is what you perceive another person doing and how you feel about it. There is a difference, for example, between saying, "You're a good girl," and saying, "It made me feel good when you went to the store for me." There is a difference between reporting your own feelings to a child and telling him or her what kind of person he or she "is." The child seen simply as "good" by the parents may come to feel loved for what he *seems* to be rather than what he is or feels. Every child has naughty, angry, and sexual feelings. He or she may have the fantasy that if these feelings were revealed, love would be withdrawn. A patient in analysis, an only child born to an older couple, was the apple of his parents' eyes. He won the outstanding student award of his first-rate prep school and went on to scholastic and extracurricular honors at an Ivy League university. After completion of graduate school, he was asked to remain on the faculty. He was superficially popular, but had had only one close friend since childhood. His self-esteem was very low. He had always been what his parents wanted him to be and felt loved and approved by them, but not really known and deeply accepted for himself. Internalization of appreciation is important to the development of the "benevolent superego," which leads to self-appreciation as contrasted to the internalization of punishment in the "punitive superego," which leads to guilt. Likewise, being identified as good or bad plays a strong role in self-identification and can be introjected as an imperative or command. The criminal may have been one always told he was bad, just like his no-good Uncle Harry. Yet simplistic praise of a person may do disservice to the totality of the developing individual.

Appreciation that comes from feelings, from inside, is different from praising or evaluating or labeling the behavior of another as good or bad. It is important and rewarding for a child to know that he can have impact, that he can do things that make others feel good. Parents need help the child gain the ability to appraise himself and to be pleased with himself. If they continually provide evaluation, either in criticism or praise (or implied criticism by withholding praise), the child has much less opportunity for providing himself with his personal evaluation. If some of his behaviors make others happy and some do not, he needs to know; he does not need to be labeled as being a good or a bad person. It is much more realistic for him to see his behavior as sometimes producing pain and sometimes producing pleasure in others. If he does not get into the habit of labeling himself as generally good or generally bad, he is on firmer ground, for obviously he is not always good, nor is he always bad.

### Allowing a Child
### the Opportunity to Fail

In a similar vein, it is not always in a child's best interest to constantly help him to solve his problems. It is easy when a child is in either physical or psychological distress to rush to his aid, to comfort his pain, to put on a Band-Aid or to help solve his problems so as to make life more pleasant and easier for him. A son or daughter struggling to solve a math problem may be better left alone for a time than given a quick answer. A father, arriving home, saw his son trying to put the inner tube back into the tire as he had seen his father do it a dozen times. He was obviously frustrated, the sweat poured off his brow, and the screwdriver constantly slipped out of his hands. The father, witnessing his plight, held himself back from jumping in and finishing the job for the son and said with concern, "It sure is tough getting that tube in, isn't it, son?" The son responded with pride, "Sure is, Dad, but I already did the front."

A vignette further illustrates the psychogenesis of strength through mastery. A septuagenarian philanthropist who had made, lost, and remade several fortunes and who was noted for his business daring and acumen as well as for his generosity, was musing at dinner with friends about his childhood in the lower East Side of New York after the turn of the century. "The turning point in my life was at age eight." His father had died when he was two; his mother struggled to survive as a piecework seamstress. At eight, out of sheer necessity, he began to peddle newspapers on a street corner. A gang of older boys demanded a percentage of his take for "protection" because he worked in their "territory." The boy refused. He was badly beaten and his left ankle broken. At City Hospital, a series of medical mishaps occurred, and repeated surgery and prolonged hospitalization were required. A permanent limp resulted. After six months in the hospital, the boy returned to the same corner and never paid the tribute—"the turning point." When asked what it was that made him *able* to go back, he pondered a moment and replied, "I guess it was my Mama. She said, 'Morris, you can do it.' " To editorialize, this expression of confidence in Morris' ability and courage represented a marked contrast to the alternative responses: the demanding and coercive, "You little coward, get the hell out there or I'll tan your fanny!" the overprotective, "Oh, my darling baby, stay here, and we'll manage somehow!" or the role-usurping, "I'll go down with you with a baseball bat, and they'll reckon with me if they try anything again." It is a task requiring sensitivity and empathy with one's child to know when he will be strengthened by attempting a difficult task or when he will be overwhelmed by something too difficult to handle.

## *Your Child's Friends*

Relationships outside the parental home are crucial to the development of strength. Possessive and competitive parents often undermine the establishment of peer relationships. "Johnnie is too rough for you to play with." "That Mary's hair always looks like a rat's nest." A child's friends need to be made to feel comfortable and welcome in the home. A child needs to be proud to show off his parents to his friends and vice versa. A child may choose to be a loner rather than risk the development of friendships that cannot be brought into his family life. The opportunity for developing interpersonal skills is often thus lost at a critical time, making it difficult in later life to form friendships. Conversely, parents in our culture may pressure a child to be "popular," making a necessity of superficial social skills, rather than fostering the joy of friendship stemming from a child's natural affection for others. The child should have wide latitude in choosing his own friends as long as the friends do not impinge on the rights and property of the parents.

### Your Child's Interests

Remembering that a child grows from the inside out, it is sometimes difficult to allow a child to develop his own interests, hobbies, and activities. Many of us have secret dreams and hopes for our children; it is not uncommon for a parent to want to live vicariously through his or her child. A drab mother may push a pretty daughter into dating and social activity in order to live vicariously through the daughter the sexual and social thrills that she missed when she was young. Everyone knows of a father who expects his son to be a great athlete. He had been an All-American half-back in college and expects his son to carry on the tradition even though the son prefers painting and pottery work. Even more malignant may be the desires of the father who could not himself become the half-back. Self-actualization is not translated other-actualization. A child must actualize himself in his lifetime, not try to fulfill the dream of his parents. Choices can be offered to a child, experiences provided, and sports or social life made possible, but if these are the only roads to parental appreciation and attention, then no other alternatives are really being made possible.

### Allowing Choosing

A strong person is able to exercise choice. Choosing is a skill developed in childhood by having parents who frequently offer choices. "Which shirt would you like to wear today?" "What would you like to have for lunch that won't be too much trouble to fix?" "Shall we go to the Doggie Diner or Gino's?" "Which babysitter would you like me to call for tomorrow night?" "Which story would you like to have me read to you?" and so on. The more choices allowed a youngster, the more he will learn how to search his inner being for his own preferences, the more he will feel that his tastes and ideas and choices count for something, and the more inner-directed he will be. By having more opportunity to please himself, he will know how to make choices relevant to his own needs. As he becomes accustomed to coming up with his own preferences, he will be developing a sense of independence and of his own individuality as an expression of his own wishes and desires rather than behaving as an extension of his father's or mother's wishes for him.

One of the most difficult tasks for a parent is to allow a child to become independent and separate, and not to control his thoughts, tastes, preferences, relationships, and values. Only through being a consistent, visible model of their own tastes, values and preferences can parents significantly influence a child to become like them. Children can become just like their parents, or like mirror images of them. An authoritarian father may create a son who rebels and later becomes rigidly permissive with his own son. His son, in turn rebelling against pervasive permissiveness, may be authoritarian with *his* son—so that grandson is like grandfather. The father and son may be basically alike although, in this case, they give different expression to their sameness—namely, their rigidity and conflicts about authority. The strong parents, who do not try to mold their sons or daughters but rather are interested in helping them know what they feel, like, and value and who help the children to be aware of these feelings, are more likely to produce integrated offspring. Such children build from within, integrate choices with preferences, and thus more likely become strong adults who will, in turn, pass this same understanding on to their sons or daughters.

### "Make-or-Break" Experiences

Obviously, strong people are not always the product of strong parents. It has already been pointed out how some of the strongest arise from the most difficult backgrounds. Some otherwise strong persons may fail to develop strength in their children, who become excessively dependent, feel inferior to their parents, or somehow fail to identify. A strong person who is the product of a bad home somehow made a break, somehow freed himself, found positive influences outside the home and discovered resources in himself. As pointed out, difficult situations during development make or break. Unfortunately, they more often break than make. It is an important but hard-to-answer question as to what enables the potentially strong to escape from or to master potentially destructive circumstances.

An outstanding young physician, who is a good husband and loving parent, grew up in an urban ghetto. His irresponsible, self-centered father, who earned a pittance through prize-fighting and posing for pornographic pictures, gambled away their miserable little house. His 350-pound mother stayed in bed all day eating ice cream. The first time he went away to a camp for underprivileged children, his parents failed to meet him at the station upon his return, and he was lost for a couple of days. However, he had intelligence, good looks, and athletic skill "going for him." He was consistently the best camper at the underprivileged children's camp and went on to become one of its counselors. When he wanted to go on to college, his father called him a lazy lout who wouldn't go out to work and refused to give him even the bus fare. His slum-school teachers banded together to raise a fund to send him through college. He had gained the love and respect of important adults outside the home.

### The Necessity for Crisis Resolution

A strong person does not distort the present in terms of the past. He is capable of living in the present, with his energies relatively available for use in the current moment. To allow a child to live in the present, it is helpful to conceive of him as passing through a series of developmental tasks relatively common to all children, in addition to experiencing other life crises unique to his own life. Heinz Wolff states:

> Some stressful experiences have a special quality and may under certain circumstances lead to personality growth; they are referred to as crisis situations, and attention has been drawn to their importance in relation to mental health and illness. Crises occur in response to sudden and more or less unexpected external threats or emotional hazards; the individual concerned experiences acute distress and is unsure whether or not he can master the new situation. He will mobilize his resources and attempt a variety of possible solutions but discovers that his customary modes of coping and reacting are inadequate; he may therefore begin to search for new solutions, and if he succeeds and the crisis is resolved, he is left with a newly discovered potential. Successful crisis resolution thus leads to increased strength and personal growth, whilst failure to resolve it leads to restriction of the personality and hold-ups in development or to actual breakdown and illness. Some of this fits in well with the definition of crisis in the Oxford Dictionary, which describes it as a "turning point" or "a state of affairs in which a decisive change for better or worse is imminent."

Wolff goes on to paraphrase Erik Erikson:

> the developing child passes through successive crises in terms of basic trust versus mistrust; autonomy versus submission associated with shame and doubt; personal initiative versus fear of disapproval and guilt; leading up to the adolescent crisis of identity formation versus identity diffusion; or the development of a negative identity based on opposition and rebellion but not yet on the choice of an identity truly one's own. Each successive crisis, if successfully lived through, leaves the individual more capable of making a satisfactory personal choice at the

next stage, and hence ultimately in adolescence when identity formation becomes the central issue.

Many crises crucial to growth are intrinsic to development. Each child must pass from a stage of total dependency to autonomy, and to an ability to respond to the needs of others. As pointed out, basic trust arises from a reliable, predictable and need-meeting early environment. Struggles over submission and socialization begin with bowel and bladder control. Masteries of a sense of time in terms of past, present, and future, and locomotion and language acquisition occur during the toddler phase. The beginning of sexual strivings and peer-group relationships follow. As Joseph Solomon points out, specific character traits such as patience, generosity, creativity, pride assertion, courage, and group loyalty arise around mastery of such developmental tasks and ensue in the mature ego. Neurotic ego traits arise from conflict and attempts at defensive or reparative secondary mastery and integration and lead to such traits as dependency, insatiability, greed, apathy, defiance, obstinacy, procrastination, appeasement, compliance, hyperactivity, bravado, jealousy, and so forth.

Other crises are unique to each child. He develops rheumatic fever, and enforced prolonged bed rest ensues; parents are divorced; twin siblings requiring much of mother's attention are born, and so forth. Again, each specific crisis provides the opportunity for new masteries or for new defeats. The wise parent realizes the regressive and progressive implications of developmental and fortuitive crises and offers support and understanding in aiding the developing child in their mastery. When the crises of growing up have been overcome and worked through, the adult is free to live in the present, relatively free from overprintings of the past. We disagree with Freud's seeing normal maturation in part as the result of repression. For example, Oedipal strivings are not repressed in the healthy child—they are given up: "To heck with Mom—I'll get my own girl some day."

### Growth in Adolescence

Adolescence is a critical time in a child's development, a time when he must begin to shape a sense of identity, confront greater financial and physical independence from his parents, a time when he or she may be confronting romance. Adolescence is often a time when the child greatly needs the support of the parents, yet also greatly needs to become more independent from them. It is also the time when most parents try to exert the most authority over their children. There is no question of their authority when the child is small. With the adolescent, parental power and authority generally are more ineffective. Some parents are permissive when their children are small, for example, but begin to fear the independence of the adolescent. Some are afraid of the adolescent's adopting friends who are not to their liking or choosing values not congruent with theirs. In an attempt to influence, they may try to coerce or force him or her to conform to their ideas of what the teenager ought to do. Gordon points out that when this occurs, adolescents do not rebel against their parents *per se,* as commonly believed, but rather they rebel against their parents' use of power. In view of the current "generation gap" between the values and world views of the young and the middle-aged, that the teen years may be times of great stress is not surprising and is evidenced by the fact that teenage suicides are increasing at an alarming rate. Families in which teenagers have attempted or succeeded in suicide have a high incidence of divorce and remarriage, new environments, new schools, death in the family, departure of brothers or sisters, or placement of the adolescent himself in a foster home or juvenile hall. Juvenile suicide studies at the University of Southern California over the past five years indicate that 72 percent of their troubled families had one or both natural parents absent from the home for various reasons. These kinds of observations once again point out the need for parents to be good models of strength and intimacy in order to facilitate the growth of strength and intimacy in their children. What a parent does really affects his child. The strong parent is deeply concerned and aware of a child's maturation.

The role of the parent does not end with the offspring's adulthood. Just as some parents never let their children grow up and still give orders to their forty-year-olds, others may throw them out on their own too soon, which may lead to premature marriage, aborted educations, and breakup of young families because of excessive realistic demands. Helpful, supportive families are long-term assets.

### Helping Kids Be Kids

So far, we have talked about helping children grow up. It is important to comment on the converse; that is, helping kids to be kids. Many parents believe that "If I treat my child as an adult, he will learn to grow up to be a mature person." The problem is that many parents, believing this, help their children to become other than children. Many a child is thus deprived of his childhood, his spontaneity, his innocence, and his playfulness by adults who insist

erceived inner and outer masteries minus the sum of
ailures; again, not only too many failures, but too few
n result in weakness. When challenges are not presently
 may need to be sought. You cannot remain complacent
essing; you can never stand still for long. If the skier never
ot learning, he is not discovering the limits of his potential.
 need in life for a certain amount of creative anxiety—
iety, enough challenge to facilitate growth and ward off
y and smugness, yet not so much as to interfere with
olvement with life.

choose new tasks, it is best to choose those that are
 rather than overwhelming. "Nothing breeds success like
an obvious truism. Continual failure also breeds failure.
eed to be chosen that have a reasonable chance of being
successfully. As you get practice at being successful, you
d at it. Too, you grow in your image of yourself as a person
cceed.

, some failures are inevitable. If there are none at all, then
ges are not great enough. It takes strength to decide to
 failure to try anew; doing so enhances strength. You can
 seeing yourself as a failure. Self-esteem should not require
t proof of success and should weather setbacks. The
of previous failures that have been overcome makes you
nafraid of new defeats. No graph of growth is a straight
s in the upward slope are unavoidable.

evelop skills in a variety of areas of life, you develop an
sense of freedom evolving from an expanded range of
greater freedom of movement from one area of life to
 you master new aspects of life, you also have more in
th a broader range of persons. Learning how to repair a
an otherwise intellectual person communicate with a
Reading *Psychology Today* might help the mechanic commu-
 a psychologist. Knowing the virtues and limitations of
s might enable a suburban matron to relate to an urban
ving competence in photography may help a parent relate
ducation can be mutual; parents can learn from their
Iany benefits accrue to those who actively seek to master
verse life tasks that are within their abilities. The sense of
 increased freedom of movement, and the increased range
rests open up many areas of communication with other

a danger in the pursuit of new masteries, however. One

that the child become "an adult." A parent can help his child be a
child by "letting his own child out to play." A parent who does not
value and allow expression to his own playfulness, innocence, and
spontaneity teaches in subtle ways, as a parental model, that these
qualities are not acceptable. The child learns quickly that it is not all
right to be a child in this sense. He learns to behave "like an adult,"
and is thus doubly handicapped. Not only is he deprived of his
childhood, in a sense, but he is not being given a model of how to
relate to his own enduring childlike qualities that are characteristic of
strong persons. Thus, the child is helped in his development by the
parental model of his own childlike (not childish) qualities.

Other parents, similarly out of touch with their own childlike
qualities, may attempt on the other hand to perpetuate the childishness of their children as a means of allowing themselves to live
vicariously. In doing this, they stunt the growth of their children and
hamper them from developing the adult-like qualities that give
balance to the freedom and spontaneity characteristic of a child.

### Valuing Your Own Growth

The strong parent is one who has progressed far enough along the
hierarchy of needs as described by Maslow that needs for love and
belongingness, esteem and self-actualization are not new and incomprehensible to him. Thus, he can value the growth and actualization
of his children, even when that growth is centered around differing
values or life styles from his own. He is encouraged, in fact, by his
children's progression beyond the traditional needs of his own
generation for security and material possessions and has compassion
for their struggles with new forms, understanding of their failures,
hopeful for their discoveries, supportive in their times of need; and he
continues to provide a source of security and stability out of which his
children can grow even when they become discouraged and insecure.
In consistently providing his children with a sense of security and a
source of love even in their struggles, he frees his children to explore
their needs for self-actualization, for personal growth, and for greater
use of their human potentials. His children may not necessarily be
successful, for success is a value more tied to those with high needs for
security and safety. His children may be looked upon as different, even
as dropouts; or they may in fact be successes, not so much out of their
needs for security as out of their own released creativity and the
discovery of their full resources as human, growing beings. It is not
that youth have different, or more, or better values than their parents

so much as that they have been released from fulfilling their lower needs to move on to filling higher ones—to actualizing. Today's youth are *building* on their parents' values rather than replacing them. A parent who in his life has had to struggle with these same issues is more apt to be understanding of this process than one who has spent much of his life meeting lower need levels.

**F**

**S**

Aspects of the development of person in all we have said so far. We hope he has been implicit, to offer some practica to grow, to bring down to earth the ab

Issues such as free will and choice a Such issues are ultimately decided righ at the present moment. You can, in f more fully human, sharing person. Ever just as much choice in trying to do bet assume that this is impossible, then yo happen and invariably nothing will ha best predictor of future behavior in a g in a similar situation, this is true becau that they can be different or because different.

The ability to control your environm to use it, all are assets that help you Being able to master skills and tasks set sense of outer mastery. As already state

a sum of
perceived
masteries c
extant, the
without re
falls, he is
There is a
enough an.
complacen·
present inv

As you
challengin;
success" is
New tasks
completed
become goo
who can su

To repea
the challer
return from
fail withou
the consta
experience
relatively
line; zigza;

As you
increasing
choices, a
another. A
common v
car helps
mechanic.
nicate wit
health foo
hippie. Ha
to a son.
children. I
new and d
mastery, th
of life inte
persons.

There i;

danger is that you may only feel worthwhile for the new accomplish-ments in your life. Another danger is that the motive for mastering new challenges may be in the pursuit of becoming a "successful" person, in the pursuit of a fantasy that will never be satisfied. The continual pursuit of newness may also reflect a fundamental boredom with yourself, a basic dislike of your inner experience, and newness for its own sake is then an escape from a barren interior. External mastery needs to be pursued in harmony and conjunction with inner mastery. External tasks are best chosen as an expression of self-consciously chosen inner values. Another danger is in being a dilettante in all areas. True fulfillment of at least one major intrinsic potential, requiring an intensity and directedness of effort, is probably necessary for most to avoid inner frustration.

### Become Comfortable with Your Anxiety

Unavoidable to growth are periods of frustration and anxiety. Frustration occurs when goal-directed behavior is thwarted. As you try to become more honest and more congruent in an interaction, as you try to master new skills, frustration is a feeling to be expected and acknowledged as it occurs. Anxiety, too, naturally accompanies venturing into unknown territory. As you attempt to be more self-aware, you will be confronting more and more parts of yourself that you may not like; for example, powerful feelings that you would just as soon not admit to yourself, let alone share with someone else. An overweight girl successfully reducing had to confront that her weight kept her from discovering that even if thin, she would feel unlovable. Very painful! As you attempt to break out of old, secure patterns of interaction, you will feel the anxiety of being insecure in a new mode of relating. You will feel more vulnerable to the rejection or aggression of others.

The same is true as you try to expand your repertoire of mastery over areas of your environment. I (JAK) decided that I was going to put in a shower at a vacation home in the Santa Cruz mountains. Never having done much plumbing, I found myself feeling an inordinate amount of anxiety. I didn't have much money to spend. Such nebulous things as traps, vents, sump holes, and the vast array of old cast iron pipe with leaded joints actually frightened me. I had no idea that alternative materials to galvanized pipe existed. I later learned that plastic pipe with bonding adhesives was very easily used. I didn't know a thing about pipe-joining compounds or "Teflon" tape to prevent leaking at joints. Faced with what appeared to be an overwhelming task, I started asking questions at hardware stores, at lumber yards, and of anyone who might know about plumbing. I managed to get the shower installed, but not without several leaks and more than a few trips back to the hardware store to have pipes recut and new questions answered. Once the job was completed, I was exhausted but my anxiety was gone. My sense of mastery and pride welled up. Gone was the anxiety of not knowing. As a matter of fact (and, admittedly, of pride) I just finished helping build my new house!

### Value the Turmoil in Your Life

Good reasons exist for temporarily accepting, even valuing turmoil or disequilibrium. One reason is that if you are, in fact, undergoing turmoil in your life, the turmoil is what you experience at the moment; it is reality for the time being. Part of being able to accept yourself is to say "It is all right, safe, and appropriate for me to feel in turmoil right now. It is not weakness to be in turmoil, but rather a natural consequence of things happening in my life. Knowing that, I will try to go about making the changes required to alter this state."

During those times of great upheaval, you are also in touch with a great breadth of feelings and experience in a way not common to everyday life, with dissonant feelings and inharmonious parts of yourself. The emotional impact of stress and upset bring these more directly into awareness. Crises are points of instability; opportunities exist for progression or for regression.

Just as it is helpful to confront or calm the distraught or frightened person, it is often helpful to challenge and "shake up" the overly complacent person. A strong person is one likely to have emerged successfully from such turmoil rather than one who has always had smooth sailing along a well-charted course. It was not until his wife left him that a successful young executive realized the central role his wife played in his life, realized his own strong dependency needs, and rediscovered the loneliness that invades the space once filled with companionship. With new vision he worked with his wife making several changes that eventually brought her home.

### Institutionalizing Personal Change

Your personal growth proceeds most smoothly as you "institutional-ize" personal change so that growth does not require major life crises or excessive turmoil. In periodically reassessing "where you are at" you avoid "getting in a rut," continuing in familiar channels just because they are comfortable. This reassessment does not mean an insatiable quest for novelty, change for its own sake, nor the abandonment of commitments. After a decade's research into the effects of stress on immunity (the body's defenses against disease), the work of my colleague and I (GFS) began to be confirmed in other laboratories, to gain acceptance and recognition. In a sense, I had it "made" and could continue with variations on the theme for a professional lifetime. In fact, I was relieved that the work would continue without me and felt free to leave for a completely different sort of work in a different setting. I really feel a sense of renewal.

### Seeking Feedback

In the service of periodic reevaluation you can seek the evaluation of others whom you respect. If you receive consistent puzzling feedback about yourself from several others, you can look within yourself to discover possible areas of your personality with which you are out of touch. A brilliant theologian saw himself as warm and loving, always reaching out, for example, yet got feedback from others that he was cold, aloof, and overly intellectual. He has since sought therapy for deeper self-exploration. In actively seeking feedback from others, he discovered in himself things beyond his own awareness. On the other hand, a strong person is sufficiently self-aware to be able to interpret and reject highly idiosyncratic feedback as representing more about the other than about himself, if such is the case.

### Accept Your "Weakness"

It is remarkable that what is most fully human is so often labeled "weak." Crying, not knowing, needing help, depending upon others, loving, hating, being conventionally "irrational," being anxious, not knowing everything, being in a state of incompleteness, needing intimacy, needing some amount of external security and stability, having fantasies—all are characteristics we all share by virtue of being human. Yet, because so much of what is distinctly human is labeled "weak," and therefore rejected or denied or feared, it is difficult for persons to own, value, and be in harmony with their full humanness. In this sense, an individual can fear and avoid essentially positive experiences, not only the negative, destructive, or noxious. Thus, in denying ourselves the possibility of having a variety of so-called "weaknesses," we tend to cut off a large part of our experience that indeed makes us most human.

Furthermore, the labeling of much of our human experience as weakness can be terribly misleading. Feelings are never appropriately labeled as being weak or strong, good or bad, rational or irrational. Feelings are real and important parts of our experience but are not governed by Aristotelian logic or moral presuppositions. To require feelings to be anything other than feelings is to ask for trouble; to require them to be rational or moral is to ask the impossible and merely sets up the mechanism for internal discord. Moral principles, operational consequences, rational considerations are brought in when feelings are dealt with, when behavior is chosen. Feelings are data—though they are not the only data used by strong persons. To acknowledge the existence of such feelings and to grant them full status as a valued part of each of our human experiences requires strength. Added courage is required to share these feelings, the full extent of our humanness, because we often must do so in the face of condemnation by others, many of whom are afraid of their own "weakness."

### Confront the Feared within Yourself

"Of all victories, first and greatest is for a man to conquer himself" (Plato). It is difficult to confront anxiety in ourselves, to accept turmoil, to acknowledge our unacceptable thoughts and fantasies. Imagine accepting and confronting fully in oneself the meaning of the fact that one is married and attracted to another person, that one has sexual feelings toward a son or daughter, that one honestly feels murderous toward a former friend by whom betrayed, that one is attracted to another of the same sex, that one considers himself liberal and humane but really feels like voting for the death penalty, that one really wants to cry when everyone expects him to "be strong," that one feels jealousy, that one feels really incompetent in an aspect of his job, that one fantasizes sexual orgies while seeing himself as good, clean-living, respectable, and religious. We all have feelings, emotions, fantasies, thoughts, and areas of "weakness" that we would just as soon not claim as being real or important parts of ourselves. These "ego-alien" aspects are often feared or cause anxiety and turmoil because they do not fit comfortably with our self-image—they are not congruent with our ego ideal. To confront them then means personal risk-taking and bringing dissonance and turmoil to ourselves. To confront all parts of ourselves means taking a risk, the risk of changing, the risk of having to grow and integrate or resolve these dissonant feelings.

Because it is difficult to gain knowledge about yourself without also undergoing personal change, it becomes clear why the rigid person— the unbending, moralistic, or authoritarian person—is not really a strong person, for he is unable to examine the full range of his experience. True strength lies in being able to look at and accept more and more of yourself. Such awareness and at-oneness does not mean to indulge in wishful fantasies, to substitute the inner for the outer, to masturbate mentally, but to use what one is to help become what one can and wishes to be.

### Come Out of Hiding

In every relationship we must weigh the risks involved and the consequences of remaining hidden and alone, but relatively secure, versus the risks and consequences of being revealed, feeling more alive and whole. Strength is required to take responsibility for your own emotions, to not "lay on" others your own hang-ups, but to share them to overcome blocks in the relationship, to gain further insight, to help achieve resolution. It is difficult to keep attitudes and feelings not aris-ing from current situations to oneself lest they be destructive to others, especially in nonintimate relationships, to recognize the difference between "letting it out with" others and "taking it out on" others.

### Select Friendships Thoughtfully

People who simply cater to your wants, disregarding their own, are but a mirror image of yourself and cannot help you grow either in your self-knowledge or in your ability to relate to others. They, in fact, are a kind of insulation cutting you off from direct contact with yourself and the outside world. You grow stronger in your independ-ence and firm sense of self in relationship to others with firm identities. You experience yourself more broadly, more fully in relationship to others who are different from you and from each other. The diversity and depth of self-knowledge parallels the diversity and depth of relatedness.

Some friends provide important links with the past; some of your present identity lies in a sense of the roots and personal history through which you have lived. Your current sense of self is bound up with the past in subtle ways. Doing things to make that past more distant, less real, does subtle damage to your current sense of self. Friends, recently divorced, made similar comments: "When I got my divorce it was like I was cut off from my past. I've had to start all over getting reacquainted with my friends, even finding out who my friends are. It's like I have to start all over telling everyone I know where I am at. And it is really disruptive. I didn't even know having a continuity of experience to the past was important until this happened."

A girl in her twenties, an adopted child, began to look for records telling her about her parents, her roots and heritage. It was important enough for her to spend several years and many fruitless trips to dead-end experiences in state and county agencies. A burden was lifted, old lines of tension faded into smiles as she returned from a trip to the state capitol where a kindly social worker finally revealed to her the nature of her origins.

### Seek Continuity of Experience

The neurotic allows distortions from the past to color the present. A strong person uses his sense of continuity with the past, his ongoing long-term relationships, and his unrepressed recollections of conflicts from the past to help prevent such distortions and to enhance his sense of personal identity.

It is a common form of rebelliousness and an act of frustration or hostility to have little or nothing to do with one's parents. Yet this kind of action is often undertaken without recognizing the value of parents as important ties with the past, providing important perspectives about how you got to be the way you are. The strong adult relates to his parents as other adults, not as he did when he was a child or adolescent. Maturity has significantly freed such a person from old conflicts to make possible new forms of relatedness. (Of course, some parents, even with help from their stronger offspring, find this shift impossible to make.)

Just as continuity of life experiences is provided through relationships with those who have shared the past, present continuity of experience or sense of wholeness comes from relationships in which one or two others touch on a broad range of current experience. Most of us feel fragmented by the way we allow ourselves to be known. We are joking with our neighbor, philosophical with our friend across town, personal with another, and relaxed with a fourth. All of these persons are important, for they bring life to different areas of ourselves that we value, areas we wish to keep alive through the touch of these significant others. But it takes someone who touches in a consistent way on the range of our experience to provide a feeling of wholeness. One must be presented wholly to be known wholly, to feel whole. Whether this wholeness is experienced in relationship to a husband or that the child become "an adult." A parent can help his child be a child by "letting his own child out to play." A parent who does not value and allow expression to his own playfulness, innocence, and spontaneity teaches in subtle ways, as a parental model, that these qualities are not acceptable. The child learns quickly that it is not all right to be a child in this sense. He learns to behave "like an adult," and is thus doubly handicapped. Not only is he deprived of his childhood, in a sense, but he is not being given a model of how to relate to his own enduring childlike qualities that are characteristic of strong persons. Thus, the child is helped in his development by the parental model of his own childlike (not childish) qualities.

Other parents, similarly out of touch with their own childlike qualities, may attempt on the other hand to perpetuate the childishness of their children as a means of allowing themselves to live vicariously. In doing this, they stunt the growth of their children and hamper them from developing the adult-like qualities that give balance to the freedom and spontaneity characteristic of a child.

### Valuing Your Own Growth

The strong parent is one who has progressed far enough along the hierarchy of needs as described by Maslow that needs for love and belongingness, esteem and self-actualization are not new and incomprehensible to him. Thus, he can value the growth and actualization of his children, even when that growth is centered around differing values or life styles from his own. He is encouraged, in fact, by his children's progression beyond the traditional needs of his own generation for security and material possessions and has compassion for their struggles with new forms, understanding of their failures, hopeful for their discoveries, supportive in their times of need; and he continues to provide a source of security and stability out of which his children can grow even when they become discouraged and insecure. In consistently providing his children with a sense of security and a source of love even in their struggles, he frees his children to explore their needs for self-actualization, for personal growth, and for greater use of their human potentials. His children may not necessarily be successful, for success is a value more tied to those with high needs for security and safety. His children may be looked upon as different, even as dropouts; or they may in fact be successes, not so much out of their needs for security as out of their own released creativity and the discovery of their full resources as human, growing beings. It is not that youth have different, or more, or better values than their parents so much as that they have been released from fulfilling their lower needs to move on to filling higher ones—to actualizing. Today's youth are *building* on their parents' values rather than replacing them. A parent who in his life has had to struggle with these same issues is more apt to be understanding of this process than one who has spent much of his life meeting lower need levels.

# 11

# FOSTERING PERSONAL STRENGTH

Aspects of the development of personal strength have been implicit in all we have said so far. We hope here to make explicit that which has been implicit, to offer some practical suggestions for those desiring to grow, to bring down to earth the abstraction of behaving strongly.

Issues such as free will and choice are not decided in the abstract. Such issues are ultimately decided right now, in the present situation, at the present moment. You can, in fact, choose right now to be a more fully human, sharing person. Even if you fail this time, you have just as much choice in trying to do better in the next moment. If you assume that this is impossible, then you will choose to make nothing happen and invariably nothing will happen. While it is true that the best predictor of future behavior in a given situation is past behavior in a similar situation, this is true because most people do not assume that they can be different or because they do not know how to be different.

### Master New Tasks

The ability to control your environment, to be in harmony with it, to use it, all are assets that help you to become a stronger person. Being able to master skills and tasks set before you allows you to feel a sense of outer mastery. As already stated, your self-image of strength is a sum of perceived inner and outer masteries minus the sum of perceived failures; again, not only too many failures, but too few masteries can result in weakness. When challenges are not presently extant, they may need to be sought. You cannot remain complacent without regressing; you can never stand still for long. If the skier never falls, he is not learning, he is not discovering the limits of his potential. There is a need in life for a certain amount of creative anxiety— enough anxiety, enough challenge to facilitate growth and ward off complacency and smugness, yet not so much as to interfere with present involvement with life.

As you choose new tasks, it is best to choose those that are challenging rather than overwhelming. "Nothing breeds success like success" is an obvious truism. Continual failure also breeds failure. New tasks need to be chosen that have a reasonable chance of being completed successfully. As you get practice at being successful, you become good at it. Too, you grow in your image of yourself as a person who can succeed.

To repeat, some failures are inevitable. If there are none at all, then the challenges are not great enough. It takes strength to decide to return from failure to try anew; doing so enhances strength. You can fail without seeing yourself as a failure. Self-esteem should not require the constant proof of success and should weather setbacks. The experience of previous failures that have been overcome makes you relatively unafraid of new defeats. No graph of growth is a straight line; zigzags in the upward slope are unavoidable.

As you develop skills in a variety of areas of life, you develop an increasing sense of freedom evolving from an expanded range of choices, a greater freedom of movement from one area of life to another. As you master new aspects of life, you also have more in common with a broader range of persons. Learning how to repair a car helps an otherwise intellectual person communicate with a mechanic. Reading *Psychology Today* might help the mechanic communicate with a psychologist. Knowing the virtues and limitations of health foods might enable a suburban matron to relate to an urban hippie. Having competence in photography may help a parent relate to a son. Education can be mutual; parents can learn from their children. Many benefits accrue to those who actively seek to master new and diverse life tasks that are within their abilities. The sense of mastery, the increased freedom of movement, and the increased range of life interests open up many areas of communication with other persons.

There is a danger in the pursuit of new masteries, however. One danger is that you may only feel worthwhile for the new accomplishments in your life. Another danger is that the motive for mastering new challenges may be in the pursuit of becoming a "successful" person, in the pursuit of a fantasy that will never be satisfied. The continual pursuit of newness may also reflect a fundamental boredom with yourself, a basic dislike of your inner experience, and newness for its own sake is then an escape from a barren interior. External mastery needs to be pursued in harmony and conjunction with inner mastery. External tasks are best chosen as an expression of self-consciously chosen inner values. Another danger is in being a dilettante in all areas. True fulfillment of at least one major intrinsic potential, requiring an intensity and directedness of effort, is probably necessary for most to avoid inner frustration.

### Become Comfortable with Your Anxiety

Unavoidable to growth are periods of frustration and anxiety. Frustration occurs when goal-directed behavior is thwarted. As you try to become more honest and more congruent in an interaction, as you try to master new skills, frustration is a feeling to be expected and acknowledged as it occurs. Anxiety, too, naturally accompanies venturing into unknown territory. As you attempt to be more self-aware, you will be confronting more and more parts of yourself that you may not like; for example, powerful feelings that you would just as soon not admit to yourself, let alone share with someone else. An overweight girl successfully reducing had to confront that her weight kept her from discovering that even if thin, she would feel unlovable. Very painful! As you attempt to break out of old, secure patterns of interaction, you will feel the anxiety of being insecure in a new mode of relating. You will feel more vulnerable to the rejection or aggression of others.

The same is true as you try to expand your repertoire of mastery over areas of your environment. I (JAK) decided that I was going to put in a shower at a vacation home in the Santa Cruz mountains. Never having done much plumbing, I found myself feeling an inordinate amount of anxiety. I didn't have much money to spend. Such nebulous things as traps, vents, sump holes, and the vast array of old cast iron pipe with leaded joints actually frightened me. I had no idea that alternative materials to galvanized pipe existed. I later learned that plastic pipe with bonding adhesives was very easily used. I didn't know a thing about pipe-joining compounds or "Teflon" tape to prevent leaking at joints. Faced with what appeared to be an overwhelming task, I started asking questions at hardware stores, at lumber yards, and of anyone who might know about plumbing. I managed to get the shower installed, but not without several leaks and more than a few trips back to the hardware store to have pipes recut and new questions answered. Once the job was completed, I was exhausted but my anxiety was gone. My sense of mastery and pride welled up. Gone was the anxiety of not knowing. As a matter of fact (and, admittedly, of pride) I just finished helping build my new house!

### Value the Turmoil in Your Life

Good reasons exist for temporarily accepting, even valuing turmoil or disequilibrium. One reason is that if you are, in fact, undergoing turmoil in your life, the turmoil is what you experience at the moment; it is reality for the time being. Part of being able to accept yourself is to say "It is all right, safe, and appropriate for me to feel in turmoil right now. It is not weakness to be in turmoil, but rather a natural consequence of things happening in my life. Knowing that, I will try to go about making the changes required to alter this state."

During those times of great upheaval, you are also in touch with a great breadth of feelings and experience in a way not common to everyday life, with dissonant feelings and inharmonious parts of yourself. The emotional impact of stress and upset bring these more directly into awareness. Crises are points of instability; opportunities exist for progression or for regression.

Just as it is helpful to confront or calm the distraught or frightened person, it is often helpful to challenge and "shake up" the overly complacent person. A strong person is one likely to have emerged successfully from such turmoil rather than one who has always had smooth sailing along a well-charted course. It was not until his wife left him that a successful young executive realized the central role his wife played in his life, realized his own strong dependency needs, and rediscovered the loneliness that invades the space once filled with companionship. With new vision he worked with his wife making several changes that eventually brought her home.

### Institutionalizing Personal Change

Your personal growth proceeds most smoothly as you "institutional-ize" personal change so that growth does not require major life crises or excessive turmoil. In periodically reassessing "where you are at" you avoid "getting in a rut," continuing in familiar channels just because they are comfortable. This reassessment does not mean an insatiable quest for novelty, change for its own sake, nor the abandonment of commitments. After a decade's research into the effects of stress on immunity (the body's defenses against disease), the work of my colleague and I (GFS) began to be confirmed in other laboratories, to gain acceptance and recognition. In a sense, I had it "made" and could continue with variations on the theme for a professional lifetime. In fact, I was relieved that the work would continue without me and felt free to leave for a completely different sort of work in a different setting. I really feel a sense of renewal.

### Seeking Feedback

In the service of periodic reevaluation you can seek the evaluation of others whom you respect. If you receive consistent puzzling feedback about yourself from several others, you can look within yourself to discover possible areas of your personality with which you are out of touch. A brilliant theologian saw himself as warm and loving, always reaching out, for example, yet got feedback from others that he was cold, aloof, and overly intellectual. He has since sought therapy for deeper self-exploration. In actively seeking feedback from others, he discovered in himself things beyond his own awareness. On the other hand, a strong person is sufficiently self-aware to be able to interpret and reject highly idiosyncratic feedback as representing more about the other than about himself, if such is the case.

### Accept Your "Weakness"

It is remarkable that what is most fully human is so often labeled "weak." Crying, not knowing, needing help, depending upon others, loving, hating, being conventionally "irrational," being anxious, not knowing everything, being in a state of incompleteness, needing intimacy, needing some amount of external security and stability, having fantasies—all are characteristics we all share by virtue of being human. Yet, because so much of what is distinctly human is labeled "weak," and therefore rejected or denied or feared, it is difficult for persons to own, value, and be in harmony with their full humanness. In this sense, an individual can fear and avoid essentially positive experiences, not only the negative, destructive, or noxious. Thus, in denying ourselves the possibility of having a variety of so-called "weaknesses," we tend to cut off a large part of our experience that indeed makes us most human.

Furthermore, the labeling of much of our human experience as weakness can be terribly misleading. Feelings are never appropriately labeled as being weak or strong, good or bad, rational or irrational. Feelings are real and important parts of our experience but are not governed by Aristotelian logic or moral presuppositions. To require feelings to be anything other than feelings is to ask for trouble; to require them to be rational or moral is to ask the impossible and merely sets up the mechanism for internal discord. Moral principles, operational consequences, rational considerations are brought in when feelings are dealt with, when behavior is chosen. Feelings are data—though they are not the only data used by strong persons. To acknowledge the existence of such feelings and to grant them full status as a valued part of each of our human experiences requires strength. Added courage is required to share these feelings, the full extent of our humanness, because we often must do so in the face of condemnation by others, many of whom are afraid of their own "weakness."

### Confront the Feared within Yourself

"Of all victories, first and greatest is for a man to conquer himself" (Plato). It is difficult to confront anxiety in ourselves, to accept turmoil, to acknowledge our unacceptable thoughts and fantasies. Imagine accepting and confronting fully in oneself the meaning of the fact that one is married and attracted to another person, that one has sexual feelings toward a son or daughter, that one honestly feels murderous toward a former friend by whom betrayed, that one is attracted to another of the same sex, that one considers himself liberal and humane but really feels like voting for the death penalty, that one really wants to cry when everyone expects him to "be strong," that one feels jealousy, that one feels really incompetent in an aspect of his job, that one fantasizes sexual orgies while seeing himself as good, clean-living, respectable, and religious. We all have feelings, emotions, fantasies, thoughts, and areas of "weakness" that we would just as soon not claim as being real or important parts of ourselves. These "ego-alien" aspects are often feared or cause anxiety and turmoil because they do not fit comfortably with our self-image—they are not congruent with our ego ideal. To confront them then means personal risk-taking and bringing dissonance and turmoil to ourselves. To confront all parts of ourselves means taking a risk, the risk of changing, the risk of having to grow and integrate or resolve these dissonant feelings.

Because it is difficult to gain knowledge about yourself without also undergoing personal change, it becomes clear why the rigid person— the unbending, moralistic, or authoritarian person—is not really a strong person, for he is unable to examine the full range of his experience. True strength lies in being able to look at and accept more and more of yourself. Such awareness and at-oneness does not mean to indulge in wishful fantasies, to substitute the inner for the outer, to masturbate mentally, but to use what one is to help become what one can and wishes to be.

### Come Out of Hiding

In every relationship we must weigh the risks involved and the consequences of remaining hidden and alone, but relatively secure, versus the risks and consequences of being revealed, feeling more alive and whole. Strength is required to take responsibility for your own emotions, to not "lay on" others your own hang-ups, but to share them to overcome blocks in the relationship, to gain further insight, to help achieve resolution. It is difficult to keep attitudes and feelings not arising from current situations to oneself lest they be destructive to others, especially in nonintimate relationships, to recognize the difference between "letting it out with" others and "taking it out on" others.

### Select Friendships Thoughtfully

People who simply cater to your wants, disregarding their own, are but a mirror image of yourself and cannot help you grow either in your self-knowledge or in your ability to relate to others. They, in fact, are a kind of insulation cutting you off from direct contact with yourself and the outside world. You grow stronger in your independence and firm sense of self in relationship to others with firm identities. You experience yourself more broadly, more fully in relationship to others who are different from you and from each other. The diversity and depth of self-knowledge parallels the diversity and depth of relatedness.

Some friends provide important links with the past; some of your present identity lies in a sense of the roots and personal history through which you have lived. Your current sense of self is bound up with the past in subtle ways. Doing things to make that past more distant, less real, does subtle damage to your current sense of self. Friends, recently divorced, made similar comments: "When I got my divorce it was like I was cut off from my past. I've had to start all over getting reacquainted with my friends, even finding out who my friends are. It's like I have to start all over telling everyone I know where I am at. And it is really disruptive. I didn't even know having a continuity of experience to the past was important until this happened."

A girl in her twenties, an adopted child, began to look for records telling her about her parents, her roots and heritage. It was important enough for her to spend several years and many fruitless trips to dead-end experiences in state and county agencies. A burden was lifted, old lines of tension faded into smiles as she returned from a trip to the state capitol where a kindly social worker finally revealed to her the nature of her origins.

### Seek Continuity of Experience

The neurotic allows distortions from the past to color the present. A strong person uses his sense of continuity with the past, his ongoing long-term relationships, and his unrepressed recollections of conflicts from the past to help prevent such distortions and to enhance his sense of personal identity.

It is a common form of rebelliousness and an act of frustration or hostility to have little or nothing to do with one's parents. Yet this kind of action is often undertaken without recognizing the value of parents as important ties with the past, providing important perspectives about how you got to be the way you are. The strong adult relates to his parents as other adults, not as he did when he was a child or adolescent. Maturity has significantly freed such a person from old conflicts to make possible new forms of relatedness. (Of course, some parents, even with help from their stronger offspring, find this shift impossible to make.)

Just as continuity of life experiences is provided through relationships with those who have shared the past, present continuity of experience or sense of wholeness comes from relationships in which one or two others touch on a broad range of current experience. Most of us feel fragmented by the way we allow ourselves to be known. We are joking with our neighbor, philosophical with our friend across town, personal with another, and relaxed with a fourth. All of these persons are important, for they bring life to different areas of ourselves that we value, areas we wish to keep alive through the touch of these significant others. But it takes someone who touches in a consistent way on the range of our experience to provide a feeling of wholeness. One must be presented wholly to be known wholly, to feel whole. Whether this wholeness is experienced in relationship to a husband or wife, lover or friend, such a relationship is needed to tie experience together, to bring a sense of meaning to life.

### Seek Models Rather Than Idols

Try to imagine what it means to be strong by thinking of persons who embody those qualities of strength that you like. But remember that modeling after another person can be dangerous. We cannot become someone else. On the other hand, it is possible to value various traits and behaviors of another person. You may see value in being gentle as a man, or in being assertive as a woman, and with persons in mind who seem to embody these traits, give them a trial run. Then, sensing their value and benefit or lack thereof, you can judge if and how they should be integrated into your own experience. In trying out new behaviors or new modes of self-expression, ask whether you are merely imitating another's behavior or genuinely trying out new ways of being. In contemporary, complex, rapidly changing cultures no one model will do. One is unlikely to grow up today apprenticed to a blacksmith father, with a secure faith in Church and King. The parent of the same sex, no matter how functional or well-integrated, can generally serve only as a partial model nowadays. As has been pointed out, a person becomes stronger as he integrates his identity from a multiplicity of sources, a difficult task but one that leads to a sense of genuine individuality. A strong person, then, has much in common with those he admires, but is like no one else. In developing strength, appropriate identification figures are actively sought out. Useful aspects of their personalities are dissected, freed from irrelevant or inappropriate aspects, in order to serve as examples to be utilized, not aped.

### Relate to Strength in Yourself and Others

You will grow in your own strength as you come to know and appreciate the strong person within yourself and, in turn, will be more apt to appreciate and see the strength in others. The more you relate to the strength in another, the more you help that person become strong, the more respect you will have for your own strengths.

If you cannot see the value and worth of a person beyond his unacceptable behaviors, if you cannot relate to his potential for strength, you will not be able to help him change and grow. He will develop to become more fully what others relate to most in him.

A Biblical example of relating to latent strength and goodness of another is the relationship of Jesus to Mary Magdalene. He did not look at the outward facts and perceive Mary as a common street-walker. He related to her inner beauty, her basic goodness, her potentialities, perhaps her strength. Being able to see these qualities in her, even beyond her own limited perception of herself, He helped foster an outer manifestation of a previously hidden beauty. If Christ had adhered to the practices of the current "honesty cult," He would have confronted her with the "truth" about herself, seeking to change her. He would only have added further to her own self-image as a person of low worth.

### Rely on Your Inner Guidance

You become stronger as you rely less on the reinforcements or sanctions of others. Within himself, a strong person tends to be less driven by guilt, fear of inner condemnation, the "punitive superego," than by what he believes in and wants to be. He knows how to praise himself. Rewards are built-in. He can be self-reinforcing, if you will. His so-called "benevolent superego," the internalization of praise, operates more frequently than the punitive. His inner systems function even in the presence of negative sanctions, as with the B-52 pilot who refused further mass bombing missions over Hanoi. The pitcher who has a sense of satisfaction in having done his best in the face of a lost game is stronger than the one cowed by the boos of the crowd.

### Respect Your Body

The body and mind function together, the mental affecting the physiological and vice versa. A strong person has concern for what he puts into his body, what he does with it, how it functions, and how it looks. He knows it needs to be used and exercised, as does the mind. His love of his body is not narcissism, however, in which the body substitutes for relationships with others. Many otherwise strong persons neglect their bodies through their preoccupation with life tasks seen as "more important." If you are seeking to be stronger, do not neglect the physical side of life, value the beauty and development of your body. Research implicates integrity of psychological adaptation and successful defense with the adequate functioning of the body.

The psychologically strong person is far more likely than the less well-integrated to be physically strong and healthy as well. This physical health is the result of the strong person's valuing his body and giving it the care it deserves through exercise, diet, sleep, and avoidance of injurious substances and through psychophysiological mechanisms linking mental and physical balance. My (GFS) research implicates integrity of psychological adaptation and successful defense with the adequate functioning of the immunological system, the body's major defensive apparatus against physical disease, especially infections and cancer. Philosophically, it is attractive to link psychological and physiological defenses, the central nervous system, and the immunological system. Both maintain integrity and homeostasis; both relate the organism to the outside word, and both have the property of memory, learning from experience.

Recent research on biofeedback control of physiological processes is substantiating ancient observations of traditional Hindu medicine. As we grow in our self-awareness, even if necessarily through the use of technological monitoring, we may become even more able to regulate pulse, blood pressure, muscle tension, blood flow, readily to achieve the state of mental relaxation associated with meditation. As we grow in our mental strength, likely we shall grow in our health.

### Your Death

It is tempting to assume that a strong person is unafraid of death. In fact, he is less likely to be as afraid of death as many of the less strong for several reasons. He is less likely to have deep regrets about his life than most. Having created a life style to his liking, having mastered his previous developmental tasks, he is apt to have a feeling of completion or satisfaction in having lived a full life. We do not want to present an unreal and Pollyanna view of the strong person and death. Many a strong person may indeed fear death, may be angry and bitter over an impending "untimely end." Many may be so involved with life that the thought of death is filled with anguish and sadness. A remarkable and courageous woman in her mid-eighties (she led an active life for another decade) said that she had lost a great deal of respect for herself because with far advancing age she had become aware of a fear of death. Previously, she had thought she could face anything in life because she was unafraid of death.

As with previous challenges, the mystery of death may be confronted with great anxiety. What is important is not so much that one has such feelings about or reactions to death, but that one is able to acknowledge and confront them. The image has frequently been presented (based on our culturally impoverished view of strength) of the famous comedian going into an operation that carries great danger of death, admired for his "bravery" and "courage" because he was able to joke and laugh with the doctors and nurses before his operation, never losing his love of life, thinking of others, putting them at their ease. Yet the fear, anguish, dread, excitement, anticipation of challenge, extreme involvement with death went unshared. The strong person does not "put up a good front"—he or she is willing and often wants to share of his involvement with death. He does not deny or hide his reality. Elisabeth Kübler-Ross in her book *On Death and Dying* points out that for any dying person, one of the greatest needs is to talk about death with others who are close. Talking about death, confronting it, facing it, enables a person to reach a point of being at peace with himself and with death—a point of acceptance. If a strong person is afraid or anxious about death, he neither hides nor denies it. If he is at peace with death, he may want to share that also. In our culture, in which death has replaced sex as a taboo subject, a process that occurs hidden away in antiseptic hospitals, the strong person will also be found more frequently as a listener to the fears of death in others. He will not need to avoid the subject with those close to him who face imminent death or who even speculate about and wish to confront death in their daily lives.

A strong person has a further advantage in facing his actual physical death in that he is likely to have experienced and confronted aspects of death during his lifetime. Being sensitive to his own experience, he is likely to have explored in himself his response to the many "Mini-deaths" experienced by us all: the loss of a friend in death, the death of a parent or close relative, the movement of a very close friend to a faraway place, the breakup with a lover—all provide one with the death of a relationship. The loss of a special person who has been able to bring out very special untapped qualities in another brings a real loss of that person's experience of himself—a death in part. Sadness, grief, or even anger or depression may accompany such losses.

Whenever there is a significant loss, whether through death or not, mourning must take place as a process of working through. John Bowlby has delineated four phases of mourning: protest, despair, detachment, and restitution (establishment of new relationships). This process can get "hung up" in any phase, leading to chronic bitterness, sadness, or withdrawal. A strong person mourns effectively (see Freud's "Work of Mourning") and goes on. Well-meaning others may try to distract the strong person. Ours is a culture that tries to "keep the bereaved busy so that he won't be overcome with grief," that provides pain-killers and tranquilizers to prevent the experiencing of any uncomfortable feeling. Seek to understand your pain. Use your less pleasant experiences to learn about yourself, to overcome. A person who has avoided the reality of pain and suffering all of his life will be totally unprepared for death. In this respect strong persons are deviant from our culture. They are much more likely than most to have confronted pain, grief, turmoil, loss, and suffering, and much more likely to have integrated them into a meaningful comprehension of life in the context of death.

In not facing death you will have trouble in facing life:

Cowards die many times before their deaths— The valiant taste of death but once. . . . —Shakespeare: *Julius Caesar*

### *Use Mental Practice*

The thesis of Maxwell Maltz's *Psychocybernetics* is that you can practice in your imagination things that you would like to be able to do more often. You can practice public speaking, meeting new people, introducing yourself to someone who is attractive, playing a sport, and so on. Mental practice has been shown to be effective in learning many perceptual-motor skills. It is a central aspect of systematic desensitization, as described by Joseph Wolpe. In this form of therapy, a person learns first how to relax and then practices being relaxed while imagining a series of carefully graded situations progressing from those only slightly anxiety-provoking to those that are quite frightening. For example, a person afraid of heights may first practice being relaxed while imagining himself on flat ground, then on a small hill, then on top of three steps, and so on up and up until he is able to imagine himself on top of a lookout at the Grand Canyon, yet still be relaxed. The key to the mental practice is in vividly imagining the situations involved.

In terms of developing personal strength then, imagine taking strong action. Imagine telling a friend that you feel warm toward him or her. Imagine being assertive with your child, not taking him to the beach this weekend because there are things that really must get done. Imagine telling a neighbor that you need your lawnmower back, etc.! Imagine yourself acting strongly in different situations rather than simply "being" a strong person. If the situation you imagine causes considerable anxiety, back off and try a similar but less threatening situation.

To think about doing something is a way of preparing actually to do it. The more fully one imagines the situation, the more fully he is practicing behaving in that situation. This is a safe and useful way to practice becoming stronger.

### Feel Free to Be Odd or Different

When about to embark on a course of action, there are many things to consider: Is what you are doing consistent with your own wishes and values? What effects will your actions have on those close to you? What will others think? If this last question is your first, then there is a good chance that you are playing for the fans rather than for yourself.

Being strong may require you to appear somewhat odd at times, choosing to be what is an expression of yourself rather than what others would have you be. You are not free if you conform for the sake of conforming or if you rebel for the sake of rebelling; you are free if you choose to do either as a current expression of what you want. One of the hardest kinds of decisions to make is to choose to do what someone else is trying to coerce you to do. Parents and teachers may be trying to get the high school senior to cut his hair. His peers like it long. Honestly, he likes it short. It requires greater strength to have his hair cut, knowing the decision to be honest and congruent while appearing to be giving in or buckling under, than it does to resist his self-judgment. It is doubly difficult for a university administration to hear the demands of a disfranchised group of students, some of whom have perpetrated violence and destruction of university property, and in conscience realize that the demands are justified and accede to those demands while still abhorring the violence associated with the confrontation.

An outstanding professional athlete decided he wanted to give up his sports career and go to professional graduate school. After rejection by several first-rank universities, he reported feeling not only disappointment, but shame, and the wish that he had not made his plans known to others. Used to the adulation of crowds he found it hard to get away from what his "fans" thought in his personal life, even though he knew that a degree from a second-rank school would still enable him to practice a profession providing expression for the intelligence, purposiveness and human compassion that were his personal traits.

### Practice Choosing

Strength is enhanced by the ability to make decisions, by weighing alternatives without the need constantly to "double think" or to remain in perpetual ambivalence over choices. You can develop your own ability to choose by practicing choosing. Practice choosing quickly. Rather than debate over which outfit to wear to the party, look at the options and choose the one that has a slight edge even though other choices still have something to recommend them.

Recognize that every choice entails some ambivalence or there would not be any problem of making a choice. To demand certainty is a waste of time. When someone makes a request, practice saying a clear yes or a clear no; it will help you feel more decisive. A friend once said that if someone asked him to do something, unless he had something else to do or had a clear initial negative reaction, he would always say, "Sure, I'll be glad to." This is a good way in which to feel more decisive, more sure of yourself. Also, it avoids the negative consequences of continual ambivalence, which is always stressful.

As you become more trusting in your impulses and choices, it is possible to more easily make larger choices with more important consequences.

### Seek Synergy

Sören Kierkegaard said, "Purity of heart is to will one thing." Although easily stated, internal peace is becoming increasingly difficult to achieve. The proliferation of values, life styles, choices, conflicting demands, complexity, all make it more and more difficult to capture that elusive state of inner harmony and singleness of purpose, "purity of heart."

As you become more sure of "where you are at," of what you value, as your behavior and ideals become more similar, as your wants and expectations more closely match what you receive, as your feelings and your role demands are less in conflict, as work and play become less oppositional, as self-interest and others' interests are less disparate, as dissonance is reduced in these areas, you become more peaceful, more sure of yourself, more secure, less vulnerable, and more able to experience yourself as whole, as strong. Acquiring a sense of inner peace requires active searching, self-conscious reflection; it is not a passive enterprise. To increase the synergy in your life, to reduce the dissonance, several concrete things can be done.

It helps to discriminate in your own current feelings the forces operating out of the past from the feelings genuinely related to the current situation. The ability to make this kind of differentiation comes from introspection, conflict, and subsequent resolution, from sharing your feelings and talking about them long enough to understand their probable origins. After a while, you can discern those areas in life where your feelings invariably tend to be colored by past experience. The boy who lived through six years of acne starting in the eighth grade was always sensitive about his appearance, no matter how clear his complexion became. The son or daughter of alcoholic parents never felt comfortable around excessive drinking. A Chicano from a poor section of town, harassed by police all of his early life, never felt comfortable around cops.

Each of us has areas of our lives that are colored by our past. Healthy insight allows us to know that those are areas in which we cannot trust our feelings as guides. However, in areas in which we know we are secure, our feelings can be very sensitive barometers about what is worthwhile and appropriate. Dissonance in these areas is a sign of irresolution that needs to be worked out. If one has no particular problems with work or parental authority, for example, but feels an uneasiness of unclear origin around his boss, this dissonance may be a good sign that there is something the matter with the boss.

The greater the degree to which you are conscious of conflicts, which can exist on many levels, the more likely they can be resolved by deliberate means. Obviously, many conflicts are unconscious and are neurotic in origin. Such conflicts can occur on different levels, from conflicts of drive (for example, from nurturance versus growth and autonomy), through conflicts between superego (conscience) and drives (for example, morality versus sexual desire) to conflicts of identity (for example, as a tough guy versus a sensitive, artistic soul). Such conflicts may even require uncovering by psychotherapeutic intervention before they can be acted upon and resolved.

Just as unease is the indicator of internal dissonance, inner peace is an indicator that inner conflicts and disintegrated factions have been for the moment integrated. You must listen sensitively to your feelings if you are to guide yourself down a path to internal harmony. Without inner awareness, there is no other guide and you will lose the way. The underlying premise to these statements is that we will seek our highest state of being, our fullest power, if unencumbered by negative cultural teachings and self-images.

### Seek Balance: Strengthen the Deficient

Carl Jung posited several dichotomies of psychological functioning: introversion (implying a rich inner life) versus extroversion (implying sociability); thinking (cognitive skills) versus feeling (emotional richness); sensation (the scientific approach toward objective evidence) versus intuition (reacting sensitively to indefinable data); the "animus" (the masculine, assertive component) versus the "anima" (the feminine, receptive component); the "persona" (or "front" with which one faces the world) versus the "shadow" (the darkly hidden side of self). Jung never placed value judgments on one or the other component, never suggested that all strive for the same combination. What seems important to us is to have some balance, to attempt to strengthen those aspects relatively weak or absent. An intuitive poet might enrich his experience by learning something of the scientific evidence about quasars, not only by lauding the beauty of the stars.

### Glimpse the Path Ahead

Some experiences are so overwhelming, so full, so rich, so intense that they give you a new vision of yourself and your potential. Maslow has named these "peak experiences." The experience of your potential is essential for its realization. For this reason peak experiences are to be valued, meditated upon, incorporated as part of your wisdom of personal potential. A peak experience is like discovering love. Once it is experienced it is valued. Once known, it provides a greater understanding of your potential.

Nancy told of her own experience. It was clear, cool, and sunny. People could be seen on distant slopes, but she was alone on her portion of the hill. Finally throwing off constraint, taking off her ski cap to let her hair fly, she took off straight down the hill, finding herself screaming with sheer delight as she skimmed across the snow, feeling a sense of communion with the wind, the trees, the snow, the people, and herself that she had never experienced before. Typically a self-contained and aloof person, Nancy has since found herself wanting to relate to others more than before, and is finding it rewarding.

Such experiences may be fleeting, but only the cynic discounts their importance. Time is not the test of the value of an experience. During such peak experiences you are in fact more whole, more yourself, more able to see clearly. Such experiences can become powerful images guiding and often radically changing your life in positive directions.

Collectively, mankind has been presented with its own analogies of the peak experience. Of the millions of men who have lived and died on the face of the earth there have been an occasional few who have evolved far beyond what Desmond Morris describes as the "naked ape," who have allowed themselves heightened awareness, who have, for whatever reason, transcended the collective level of awareness of mankind. Such men as Jesus of Nazareth, Buddha, and others represent the potential of which we are capable if we would allow it. These men represent visions of the integrated man.

### Discern False Prophets

In our search for guides, idols, gurus, visionaries, Gods, we are beseiged by false prophets, glittering tinsel, and a host of many pseudo-gods and would-be teachers who would seek our devotion. Is the fifteen-year-old whose Astrodome appearances were billed as "the most important event since the coming of Christ" a guru or a false prophet? How does one tell a Gandhi from a Charles Manson? We suggest, in keeping with the central themes of this book, that you not look at credentials, not look at charisma, not look at training, at followers, or at miracles. Look not to what the guru does, but rather perceive what he evokes in you. The path to growth lies within your relationship to him or her. Does life become simpler, more peaceful? Are paradoxes transcended? Do you see more clearly? Do you feel more personally distinct while also developing a closer relatedness to fellow man? Growth tends to foster communion with the humanness of others rather than condescension in relationship to the unenlightened.

Not only does growth begin within, it also begins from "where you are at" and when you are ready. You may look ahead to the man on the crest of the hill who calls back of the vision of beauty lying on the other side, but you cannot immediately share the vision if you still must cross the plain, ford the river, and climb the hill. The traveler high on the hill is worth following if he helps you enjoy the plain, savor the river, relate to the hill, and thus prepare you for the beauty and the ecstasy at the top.

Beware the prophet who evokes feelings of guilt, inadequacy, and failure, whose message is that you are a sinner and have fallen short. Though guilt and shame may motivate you to action, they rarely foster growth.

Awareness does not exist in the future but in the present. Similarly, growth involves being increasingly open to your experience now. You can't find or grow from an experience that isn't there. Strength involves feeling good about yourself for growing, not chastising yourself for falling short of your ideal.

# BIBLIOGRAPHY

ADLER, A., *The Neurotic Constitution*. New York: Moffat-Yard, 1917.

———, "The practice and theory of individual psychology," in T. Shipley, *Classics in Psychology*. New York: Philosophical Library, 1961, pp. 687–714.

ALBERTI, R., and M. EMMONS, *Your Perfect Right*. San Luis Obispo, Calif.: Impact, 1970.

ALEXANDER, F., *Psychosomatic Medicine*. New York: Norton, 1950.

ALTIZER, T., and W. HAMILTON, *Radical Theology and the Death of God*. New York: Bobbs-Merrill, 1966.

AMERICAN FRIENDS SERVICE COMMITTEE, *Working Loose*. Ann Arbor, Mich.: Edward Bros., 1971.

AMKRAUT, A., and G. SOLOMON, "Stress and Murine Sarcoma Virus (Moloney)-Induced Tumors, *Cancer Research* (July 1972) 32:1428–33.

AMKRAUT, A., G. SOLOMON, M. ALLANSMITH, B. McCLELLAN, and M. RAPPAPORT, "Immunoglobulins and Improvement in Acute Schizophrenic Reactions, *Archives of General Psychiatry*, 28 (1973), 673.

ANSBACHER, H., and R. ANSBACHER, eds., *The Individual Psychology of Alfred Adler*. New York: Basic Books, 1956.

ARDREY, R., *The Territorial Imperative*. New York: Atheneum, 1966.

ARIETI, S., *The Will to be Human*. New York: Quadrangle Books, 1972.

BACH, G., and R. DEUTSCH, *Pairing*. New York: Avon Books, 1970.

BACH, G., and P. WYDEN, *The Intimate Enemy*. New York: Avon Books, 1968.

BAHNSON, C., ed., *Second Conference on Psychophysiological Aspects of Cancer.* Annual N.Y. Academy of Science, 1969, vol. 164.

BANDURA, A., and R. WALTERS, *Social Learning and Personality Development.* New York: Holt, Rinehart and Winston, 1963.

BARBER, T., L. DiCARA, J. KAMIYA, N. MILLER, D. SHAPIRO, and J. STOYVA, eds., *Biofeedback and Self-Control.* New York: Aldine Atherton, 1971.

BAY, C., *The Structure of Freedom.* Stanford, Calif.: Stanford University Press, 1958.

BEISER, M., "Assets and Affects," *Archives of General Psychiatry,* 27 (1972), 545-49.

BENEDICT, R., "Synergy: Patterns of the Good Culture," *American Anthropologist,* 72 (1970), 320-33.

BERLINER, B., "Libido and Reality in Masochism," *Psychoanalytic Quarterly,* 9 (1940), 322.

BOWLBY, J., *Attachment.* New York: Basic Books, 1969.

———, *Maternal Care and Mental Health.* Geneva: World Health Organization, 1952.

BRADBURN, N. M., *The Structure of Psychological Well-Being.* Chicago, Ill.: Aldine, 1969.

BRADBURN, N. M., and D. CAPLOVITZ, *Reports on Happiness.* Chicago, Ill.: Aldine, 1965.

BRAND, S., ed., *The Whole Earth Catalogue.* Menlo Park, Calif.: Portola Institute, 1970.

BRETALL, R., ed., *A Kierkegaard Anthology.* New York: Modern Library, 1946.

BRODERICK, C., "Man + Woman: A Consumer's Guide to Contemporary Pairing Patterns including Marriage," *Human Behavior,* 1 (1972), 8-15.

BUBER, M., *I and Thou.* New York: Charles Scribner's Sons, 1950.

BUGENTHAL, J., "Humanistic psychology: A New Breakthrough," *American Psychologist,* 18 (1963), 563-67.

BURSTEN, B., *The Manipulator.* New Haven, Conn.: Yale University Press, 1973.

BUTTON, A., *The Authentic Child.* New York: Random House, 1969.

CAMUS, A., *The Rebel,* trans. A. Bowen. New York: Vantage Books, 1956.

CASTANEDA, C., *A Separate Reality: Further Conversations with Don Juan.* New York: Simon and Schuster, 1971.

CHURCHILL, W., *Homosexual Behavior among Males.* Englewood Cliffs, N.J.: Prentice-Hall, 1967.

CLARK, L., "A Comparative View of Aggressive Behavior," *American Journal of Psychiatry,* 119 (1962), 336.

COMFORT, A., *The Joy of Sex.* New York: Crown, 1973.

COOPERSMITH, S., *Antecedents of Self-Esteem.* San Francisco, Calif.: Freeman, 1967.

————, "Studies in Self-Esteem," *Scientific American*, 218 (1968), 96–106.

DARWIN, C., *The Origin of the Species and the Descent of Man*. New York: Modern Library, 1936.

DEMENT, W., "Sleep," in K. Fisher, A. Dawe, C. Lyman, E. Schönbaum, and F. South, Jr., *Mammalian Hibernation III*. London: Oliver and Boyd, 1967.

DE UNAMUNO, M., *Tragic Sense of Life*. New York: Macmillan, 1921.

DIMSDALT, J., "The Coping Behavior of Nazi Concentration Camp Survivors," *American Journal of Psychiatry*, 131, No. 7 (1974), 792–93.

DOBZHANSKY, T., *Mankind Evolving: The Evolution of the Human Species*. New Haven, Conn.: Yale University Press, 1962.

DUBOS, R., *Man Adapting*. New Haven, Conn.: Yale University Press, 1965.

EDWARDS, T., ed., *The New Dictionary of Thoughts*. Garden City, N.Y.: Hanover House, 1963.

ELLIS, A., *Sex Without Guilt*. New York: Grove Press, 1965.

ERIKSON, E., *Childhood and Society*, 2nd ed. New York: Norton, 1969.

EYSENCK, H., "The Development of Moral Values in Children: The Contribution of Learning Theory," *British Journal of Educational Psychology*, 30 (1960), 11–22.

FAIRFIELD, R., *Communes USA*. Baltimore, Maryland: Penguin Books, 1971.

FRANK, J., *Sanity and Survival. Psychological Aspects of War and Peace*. New York: Random House, 1967.

FRANK, L., "Genetic Psychology and Its Prospects," *American Journal of Orthopsychiatry*, 21 (1951), 506.

FRANKL, V., *Man's Search for Meaning*. New York: Washington Square Press, Inc., 1963.

————, "Self-Transcendence as a Human Phenomenon," *Journal of Humanistic Psychology*, 6 (1966), 97–106.

————, *The Will to Meaning*. New York: World, 1969.

FREEMAN, L., "The Answer." CBS Studio City, Calif.: Leonard Freeman Productions, 1965.

FREUD, A., *The Ego and the Mechanisms of Defense*. New York: International University Press, 1946.

FREUD, S., "Beyond the Pleasure Principle" (1922), in *The Standard Edition of the Complete Psychological Works of Sigmund Freud*, transl. and ed. J. Strachey with others. London: Hogarth, 1955, Vol. 18, p. 7.

————, "Civilization and Its Discontents" (1930), *Standard Edition*, 1961, Vol. 21, p. 64.

FRIEDMAN, M., and R. ROSENMAN, "Coronary-Prone Individuals (Type A Behavior Pattern): Some Biochemical Characteristics," *JAMA*, 212 (1970), 1030.

FROMM, E., *The Anatomy of Human Destructiveness*. New York: Holt, Rinehart, and Winston, 1973.

FROMM, E., *The Art of Loving*. New York: Harper & Row, 1956.

————, *Escape from Freedom*. New York: Farrar and Rinehart, 1941.

————, *You Shall Be As Gods*. Greenwich, Conn.: Fawcett, 1956.

————, *Man for Himself*. New York: Rinehart, 1947.

GIBRAN, K., *Jesus: The Son of Man*. New York: Knopf, 1928.

————, *The Prophet*. New York: Knopf, 1923.

GORDON, T., *Parent Effectiveness Training*. New York: Peter H. Wyden, Inc., 1970.

GORNEY, R., *The Human Agenda*. New York: Simon and Schuster, 1972.

GREEN, R., *Sexual Identity Conflict in Children and Adults*. New York: Basic Books, 1974.

GREENACRE, P., *Trauma, Growth, and Personality*. New York: Norton, 1952.

GRINKER, R., "Normality Viewed as a System," *Archives of General Psychiatry*, 17 (1967), 682–735.

GROSS, K., *The Play of Man*. New York: D. L. Appelton, 1901.

GUNTHER, B., *What to Do Till the Messiah Comes*. New York: Macmillan, 1971.

HALL, E., *The Silent Language*. Garden City, N.Y.: Doubleday, 1959.

HARLOW, H., "Love in Infant Monkeys," *Scientific American*, 1959, 200–268.

————, "Social Deprivation in Monkeys," *Scientific American*, 1962, Nov. 1, 1.

HARRIS, T., *I'm OK—You're OK*. New York: Harper & Row, 1969.

HARTMAN, H., *Ego Psychology and the Problem of Adaptation*. New York: International Universities Press, 1958.

HARTMAN, H., E. KRIS, and R. LOEWENSTEIN, "Notes on the Theory of Aggression, in *Psychoanalytic Study of the Child*, vols. 3, 4. New York: International Universities Press, 1949.

HEDGEPETH, W., and D. STOCK, *The Alternative*. London: Collier-Macmillan, Ltd., 1970.

HEIDEGGER, M., *The Question of Being*, trans. T. Wayne. New York: Harper, 1958.

HESCHEL, A., *Who is Man?* Stanford, Calif.: Stanford University Press, 1965.

HESSE, H., *Siddartha*. New York: New Directions, 1951.

HOLLENDER, M., L. LUBORSKY, and T. SCARAMELLA, "Body Contact and Sexual Excitement," *Archives of General Psychiatry*, 20 (1969), 188.

HOLMES, T., and R. RAHE, "The Social Readjustment Rating Scale," *Journal of Psychosomatic Research*, 11 (1967), 213–18.

HORNEY, K., *Neurosis and Human Growth*. New York: Norton, 1950.

————, *New Ways in Psychoanalysis*. New York: Norton, 1939.

HOWARD, J., *Please Touch—A Guided Tour of the Human Potential Movement*. New York: McGraw-Hill, 1970.

HUA, E., *Kung Fu Meditations and Chinese Proverbial Wisdom*. Ventura, Calif.: Parout Press, 1973.

HUBBARD, L., *When in Doubt, Communicate.* Ann Arbor, Mich.: Scientology, 1969.

————, *The Problems of Work.* Edinburgh, Scotland: The Publishers Organization World Wide, 1967.

HUNT, M., *The Affair.* New York: The New American Library, 1969.

HUXLEY, L., *You Are Not the Target.* Hollywood, Calif.: Wilshire Book Co., 1963.

ILLICH, I., *Deschooling Society.* New York: Harper & Row, 1970.

"J.," *The Sensuous Woman.* New York: Dell, 1969.

JAMES, M., and D. JONGEWARD, *Born to Win.* Menlo Park, Calif.: Addison-Wesley, 1971.

JANOUSKY, D., M. EL-YOUSEF, J. DAVIS and H. SERKERKE, "A Cholenergic-Adrenergic Hypothesis of Mania and Depression," *Lancet* (September 1972), pp. 632–35.

JOHNSON, A., and S. SZUREK, "The Genesis of Antisocial Acting Out in Children and Adults," *Psychoanalytic Quarterly,* 21 (1952), 323.

JOURARD, S., *Disclosing Man to Himself.* New York: Van Nostrand, 1968.

————, *The Transparent Self.* New York: Van Nostrand Reinhold, 1971.

JUNG, C., *Man and His Symbols.* Garden City, N.Y.: Doubleday, 1964.

————, *Memories, Dreams, and Reflections.* New York: Pantheon, 1961.

KAHN, H., and B. BRUCE-BRIGGS, *Things to Come: Thinking about the 70's and 80's.* New York: Macmillan, 1972.

KANGAS, J., "Group Member's Self-Disclosure as a Function of Preceding Self-Disclosure by Leader or Other Group Member," *Comparative Group Studies* (February 1971), 65–70.

KAPLAN, H., "History and Theoretical Concepts of Psychophysiologic Medicine," *Psychiat. Annals,* 42 (1973), 12.

KATZ, E., *Armed Love.* New York: Bantam, 1973.

KAZAN, E., *The Arrangement.* New York: Avon, 1972.

KENISTON, K., *The Uncommitted; Alienated Youth in American Society.* New York: Harcourt, Brace & World, 1965.

————, *Young Radicals.* New York: Harcourt, Brace & World, 1968.

KENNEDY, J., *Profiles in Courage.* New York: Pocket Books, 1956.

KIERKEGAARD, S., *Fear and Trembling.* Princeton, N.J.: Princeton University Press, 1941.

KINSEY, A., W. POMEROY and C. MARTIN, *Sexual Behavior in the Human Male.* Philadelphia: Saunders, 1948.

————, *Sexual Behavior in the Human Female.* Philadelphia: Saunders, 1953.

KOESTLER, A., *The Act of Creation.* New York: Macmillan, 1964.

KOHLBERG, L., "The Development of Children's Orientations toward Moral

Order: II Social Experience, Social Conduct, and the Development of Moral Thought. *Vita Humana*, Basel, 1964.

KOPP, S., *If You Meet the Buddha on the Road, Kill Him!*, Ben Lomond, Calif.: Science and Behavior Books, 1972.

KÜBLER-ROSS, E., *On Death and Dying*. New York: Macmillan, 1970.

LAING, R., *The Divided Self.* London: Tavistock, 1960.

————, *Knots*. New York: Random House, 1970.

————, *The Politics of Experience*. New York: Pantheon, 1968.

LAIR, J., *I Ain't Much, Baby—But I'm All I've Got*. Garden City, N.Y.: Doubleday, 1972.

LEE, S., ed., *Thor, Captain America, Iron Man, Marven Triple Action*. New York: Magazine Management Co., December 8, 1972.

LeSHAN, L., and R. WORTHINGTON, "Personality as a Pathogenesis of Cancer: Review of Literature," *British Journal of Medical Psychology*, 29 (1956), 49.

LEVENSON, E., *The Fallacy of Understanding. An Inquiry into the Changing Structure of Psychoanalysis*. New York: Basic Books, 1972.

LEVINE, M., *Psychiatry and Ethics*. New York: George Braziller, 1972.

LIFTON, R., *Home from the War*. New York: Simon & Schuster, 1973.

LORENZ, K., *On Aggression*. New York: Harcourt, Brace & World, 1966.

LOWEN, A., *The Betrayal of the Body*. New York: Collier, 1967.

McCAFFREY, J., ed., *The Homosexual Dialectic*. Englewood Cliffs, N.J.: Prentice-Hall, 1972.

McLUHAN, M., *Understanding Media: The Extension of Man*. New York: McGraw-Hill, 1969.

McREYNOLDS, P., "Exploratory Behavior: A Theoretical Interpretation," *Psychological Reports*, 11 (1962), 311.

MALTZ, M., *Psycho-Cybernetics*. Hollywood, Calif.: Wilshire, 1965.

MASLOW, A., *The Farther Reaches of Human Nature*. New York: Viking, 1971.

————, *Motivation and Personality*. New York: Harper & Row, 1954.

————, *Religions, Values, and Peak Experiences*. Columbus, Ohio: Ohio State University Press, 1964.

————, *Toward a Psychology of Being*. Princeton, N.J.: Van Nostrand, 1962.

MAY, R., *Love and Will*. New York: Norton, 1969.

————, *Power and Innocence*. New York: Norton, 1972.

MENNINGER, K., *The Crime of Punishment*. New York: Viking, 1968.

————, *The Vital Balance*. New York: Viking, 1963.

MENNINGER, R., "Decisions in Sexuality: An Act of Impulse, Conscience or Society?" *Medical Aspects of Human Sexuality* (June 1974), pp. 56–80.

MILLS, R., *Young Outsiders, A Study in Alternative Communities*. New York: Pantheon, 1973.

MITCHNER, J., *The Drifters*. Greenwich, Conn.: Fawcett, 1971.

MONTAGU, A., *Touching.* New York: Harper & Row, 1971.

MONTAGUE, M., *Man and Aggression.* New York: Oxford University Press, 1968.

MORRIS, D., *The Human Zoo.* New York: McGraw-Hill, 1969.

———, *Intimate Behavior.* New York: Random House, 1971.

MOUSTAKAS, C., *The Authentic Teacher.* Cambridge, Mass.: Howard A. Doyle, 1966.

———, *Loneliness.* Englewood Cliffs, N.J.: Prentice-Hall, 1961.

———, *Loneliness and Love.* Englewood Cliffs, N.J.: Prentice-Hall, 1972.

———, *Personal Growth.* Cambridge, Mass.: Howard A. Doyle, 1971.

MOWRER, O., *The New Group Therapy.* New York: Van Nostrand Reinhold, 1964.

MURPHY, M., *Golf in the Kingdom.* New York: Viking, 1972.

NEUBECK, G., ed., *Extramarital Relations.* Englewood Cliffs, N.J.: Prentice-Hall, 1969.

O'NEILL, N., and G. O'NEILL, *Open Marriage.* New York: M. Evans and Company, 1972.

ORROCK, R., "You Must Go Home Again," *Catholic Voice*, Nov. 23, 1972.

OVESEY, L., *Homosexuality and Pseudohomosexuality.* New York: Science House, 1969.

PACKARD, V., *Nation of Strangers.* New York: McKay, 1972.

PARSONS, T., "Definitions of Health and Illness in the Light of American Values and Social Structure," in E. Jaco, ed., *Patients, Physicians, and Illness.* New York: Free Press, 1958.

PLATO, *The Symposium*, trans. W. Hamilton. Baltimore: Penguin, 1951.

RAHE, R., "Life Crisis and Health Change," in C. Thomas, *Psychotropic Drug Response: Advances in Prediction.* Springfield, Ill.: Thomas, 1969.

RATTREY-TAYLOR, B., *Rethink: A Paraprimitive Solution.* New York: Dutton, 1973.

RICHTER, D., "The Biological Investigation of Schizophrenia," *Biological Psychiatry*, 2 (1970), 153.

RIESMAN, D., *The Lonely Crowd.* New Haven, Conn.: Yale University Press, 1950.

RIMMER, R., *The Harrad Experiment.* New York: Bantam, 1966.

———, *Proposition 31.* New York: New American Library, 1968.

———, *The Rebellion of Yale Marratt.* Boston: Challenge Press, 1964.

ROGERS, C., *Becoming Partners: Marriage and Its Alternatives.* New York: Delacorte, 1971.

———, *On Becoming a Person.* Boston: Houghton Mifflin, 1961.

ROSENFELS, P., *Homosexuality: The Psychology of the Creative Process.* New York: Libra, 1971.

RUBIN, T., *The Angry Book*. New York: Collier, 1969.

SALK, J., *The Survival of the Wisest*. New York: Harper & Row, 1973.

SARTRE, J., *Being and Nothingness*, trans. H. BARNES. New York: Washington Square Press, 1956.

SEARS, R., E. MACCOBY, and H. LEVIN, *Patterns of Child Rearing*. Evanston, Ill.: Row, Peterson, 1957.

SEEMAN, J., "Toward a Concept of Personality Integration," *American Psychologist*, 14 (1959), 633–37.

SHOBEN, E., "Toward a Concept of the Normal Person," *American Psychologist*, 12 (1957), 183–89.

SILVERBERG, W., *Childhood Experience and Personal Destiny*. New York: Springer, 1952.

SIMONS, J., and J. REIDY, *The Risk of Loving*. New York: Herder and Herder, 1968.

SIMPSON, G., *The Meaning of Evolution*. New Haven, Conn.: Yale University Press, 1949.

SIU, R., *The Man of Many Qualities: A Legacy of the I Ching*. Cambridge, Mass.: MIT Press, 1968.

SKINNER, B., *Beyond Freedom and Dignity*. New York: Knopf, 1971.

SOLOMON, G., "Psychiatric Casualities of the Vietnam Conflict with Particular Reference to the Problem of Heroin Addiction," *Modern Medicine*, September 1971, 119–201, 211, and 215.

———, "Psychodynamic Aspects of Aggression," in D. Daniels et al., eds., *Violence and the Struggle for Existence*. New York: Little, Brown, 1970.

———, Psychophysiological Aspects of Rheumatoid Arthritis and Autoimmune Disease," in O. Hill, *Modern Trends in Psychosomatic Medicine 2*. London: Butterworth, 1970.

SOLOMON, G., and A. AMKRAUT, "Emotions, Stress and Immunity," *Frontiers of Radiation Therapy and Oncology*, 7, 84–96. Baltimore: University Park Press, 1972.

SOLOMON, G., and R. MOOS, "The Relationship of Personality to the Presence of Rheumatoid Factor in Asymptomatic Relatives of Patients with Rheumatoid Arthritis," *Psychosomatic Medicine*, 27 (1965), 350.

SOLOMON G., V. ZARCONE, JR., R. YOERG, N. SCOTT, and R. MAURER, "Three Psychiatric Casualties from Vietnam," *Archives of General Psychiatry*, 25 (1971), 522–24.

SOLOMON, J., "Alice and the Red King: the Psycho-analytic View of Existence," *International Journal of Psycho-Analysis*, 44 (1963), 63–73.

———, "The Fixed Idea as an Internalized Transitional Object," *American Journal of Psychotherapy*, 16, No. 4 (1962), 632.

———, *A Synthesis of Human Behavior*. New York: Grune and Stratton, 1954.

STEINER, G. (E. HALL interviewer), "The Freakish Passion," *Psychology Today*, 6 (1973), 57–69.

STOLLER, R., "The 'Bedrock' of Masculinity and Femininity: Bisexuality," *Archives of General Psychiatry*, 26 (1972), 207-12.

———, "Overview: The Impact of New Advances in Sex Research on Psychoanalytic Theory," *The American Journal of Psychiatry*, 130 (1973), 3, 241-51.

STORR, A. *Human Aggression.* New York: Atheneum, 1968.

———, *Human Destructiveness.* New York: Basic Books, 1972.

SZASZ, T., *The Myth of Mental Illness: Foundation of a Theory of Personal Conduct.* New York: Hoeber-Harper, 1961.

TEICHER, J., "The Alienated, Older, Isolated Male Adolescent," *American Journal of Psychotherapy*, 26, No. 3 (1972), 401-7.

TEILHARD DE CHARDIN, P., *The Future of Man*, trans. M. DENN. New York: Harper & Row, 1964.

———, *The Phenomenon of Man.* New York: Harper & Row, 1959.

TIGER, L., *Men in Groups.* New York: Random House, 1969.

TILLICH, P., *The Courage to Be.* New Haven, Conn.: Yale University Press, 1952.

TOFFLER, A., *Future Shock.* New York: Random House, 1970.

TOURNIER, P., *The Strong and the Weak*, trans. E. HUDSON. Philadelphia: Westminster Press, 1948.

TRILLING, L., *Sincerity and Authenticity.* Cambridge, Mass.: Harvard University Press, 1972.

TRUNGPA, C., *Meditation in Action.* Berkeley, Calif.: Shanbula Publications, 1969.

VALLIANT, G., "Natural History of Male Psychological Health: II. "Some Antecedents of Healthy Adult Adjustment," *Archives of General Psychiatry*, 31 (1974), 15-22.

VILAR, E., *The Manipulated Man.* New York: Farrar, Straus & Giroux, 1973.

WATSON, R., *Psychology of the Child.* New York: Wiley & Sons, 1960.

WATTS, A., *Psychotherapy East and West.* New York: Pantheon, 1961.

WEINCHEL, E., "The Ego in Health and Normality," *Journal of the American Psychoanalytic Association*, 18 (1970), 682-735.

WHEELIS, A., *How People Change.* New York: Harper & Row, 1973.

———, *The Moralist*, New York: Basic Books, 1973.

WHITE, R., *The Abnormal Personality.* New York: Ronald, 1964.

———, "Competence and the Growth of Personality," in J. Masserman, ed., *Science and Psychoanalysis. Vol. XI. The Ego*, 42-58. New York: Grune & Stratton, 1967.

WHORF, B., *Science and Linguistics.* The Technology Review, 42: No. 6 (1940).

WHYTE, W., *The Organization Man.* New York: Simon & Schuster, 1956.

WINNICOTT, D., "Transitional Objects and Transitional Phenomena," *International Journal of Psycho-analysis*, 34 (1953), 89.

WOLFE, T., *The Hills Beyond.* New York: Harper & Brothers, 1941.

WOLFF, H., "Crisis Points and Problems of Identity," *Journal of Psychosomatic Research,* 16 (1972), 229–34.

WOLPE, J., *Psychotherapy by Reciprocal Inhibition.* Stanford, Calif.: Stanford University Press, 1958.

YALOM, I., *Encounter Groups: First Facts.* New York: Basic Books, 1973.

————, *The Theory and Practice of Group Psychotherapy.* New York: Basic Books, 1970.

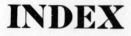

# INDEX